Behind the Smile

Behind the Smile

My Journey out of Postpartum Depression

Marie Osmond

WITH **Marcia Wilkie** AND **Dr. Judith Moore**

WARNER BOOKS

A Time Warner Company

Warner Books, Inc., 1271 Avenue of the Americas, New York, NY 10020
Visit our Web site at www.twbookmark.com
🐦 A Time Warner Company

Printed in the United States of America

First Printing: May 2001
10 9 8 7 6 5 4 3 2 1

Library of Congress Cataloging-in-Publication Data

Osmond, Marie, 1959–
    Behind the smile : my journey out of postpartum depression / Marie Osmond
with Marcia Wilkie and Judith Moore.
        p. cm.
    Includes bibliographical references.
    ISBN 0-446-52776-9
    I. Osmond, Marie, 1959—Health.   2. Postpartum depression—Patients—
Biography.   I. Wilkie, Marcia.   II. Moore, Judith, Dr.   III. Title.

    RG852.O84 2001
    362.1'9876—dc21
    [B]   2001017796

Text design by Stanley S. Drate/Folio Graphics Co. Inc.

To my mother, for giving me life
and the courage to live it more fully.

◆

And to all the women enduring PPD
who shared their stories with me; a promise kept.

Contents

Acknowledgments

There's a side effect of postpartum depression that I chose not to mention in the book because I felt the best place for it to be revealed is here in the thank-yous. It's one that I hope to live with for the rest of my life—immeasurable gratitude. When I was barely existing with PPD, every act of kindness both large and small was magnified for me. Each act felt like a hand to hold in the darkness and a guide to show me a way to get through the next minute, hour, and day.

There are many who deserve my gratitude. I especially want to thank those who made this book a possibility.

My husband, Brian, for his immeasurable love and for encouraging me to tell my story truthfully, and my children, who make me love being a mother more every day. You are and will always be everything to me.

My mother and father, Olive and George Osmond, and all my brothers: I live with your love and support every day. What a fortunate person I am.

Dr. Judith Moore: You are a healer in the truest sense of the word. Thank you for being dedicated to this project and to the many women who will benefit from your knowledge.

Marcia Wilkie: I love our friendship. Your untiring efforts through countless hours of interviews, having my babies hanging off your limbs, long plane trips, doll signings, two A.M. IHOP emergencies, and just thinking out loud with me brought my thoughts, my experiences, and this book together. I couldn't have done it without you.

My business associates, who are also my friends: Karl Engemann, my personal manager, because you held me together in my most scattered moments, and for your loving protection throughout. Allen Finlinson, my business manager, for arranging and rearranging my schedule and for being smart enough to keep my calendar in pencil. Steve Horton, my CPA and business adviser, for your assistance and support, and for bringing in extra-crispy bacon (just the way I like it) when we had been up all night writing. Lisa Hatch, my creative director, for your excellent editing eye, the hundreds of laughs, and your willingness to listen again and again. Kesti White, for formatting, fixing, and finding where I left my glasses, my keys, my notes, and my brain.

Also, thank you to those who stood by me when I could barely stand on my own, and who filled in the blanks when I forgot: Missy Garcia, for your loving friendship and steady presence, for pulling my hand out of the box of chocolates after three pieces, and for giving me directions to work almost every day! Georgia Blosil and Kathy Blosil, I'm so grateful for family. Patty Leoni, my lifelong true-blue partner in crime, I love you. LuAnn and Mike Samuelian, Shawn King, Linda Glather, Charles Cook, Maureen FitzPatrick, Dina Cerchione, Ret Turner, Leslie Feinauer, Maria Seno, Kim Auten, and the staff and crew of *Donny & Marie*.

Finally, many thanks to Mel Berger and John Ferriter at the William Morris Agency, Marleah Leslie and Anne Israel-Gurrola, Caryn Karmatz Rudy, Amy Einhorn, and Molly Chehak at Warner Books.

Marcia Wilkie extends sincere thanks to Lizzie Isely, Elizabeth Lachman, Maureen FitzPatrick, and especially to Patricia Bechdolt.

Behind the Smile

Introduction

———◆———

This weekend is my son Matthew's first birthday. Giving birth to him put me on a new course in life. It opened my eyes to many things in my personal life that needed renewal or change and made me aware of the lives of many, many women who struggle, as I have, with postpartum depression. He sure accomplished a lot in his first year of life.

Seventeen years ago, when I went into the hospital to deliver my first baby, my mother said to me, "Don't worry, Marie. The pain will only get so bad and then you will just black out." I've always appreciated my mother's willingness to tell me the truth about life in her humorous way (it's where I got my own sense of humor). However, in my experiences of giving birth, I was never able to just "black out." I guess there's a downside to having a high pain tolerance. But even that wasn't enough to deal with the pain brought on by postpartum depression. Still, I couldn't just black out. I had to experience it in full. Now I know there was a reason.

Postpartum depression (PPD) is a heartless invader that holds over 15 percent of new mothers hostage. It floods them with self-doubt, anxiety, and feelings of shame that can lead to isolation. It can occur right after giving birth, or weeks and even months later. It can happen after any birth, not just the first baby. It's estimated that 80 percent of all new mothers have a short-term experience with the "blues" due to fluctuating postnatal hormones, however, women with PPD have a much more severe and lasting reaction. It may begin with a hormonal and chemical imbalance, but the effects on emotions, moods, and behavior last well beyond the two weeks considered normal for the baby blues. Some women continue to experience PPD for up to two years after the birth of a baby. Adoptive mothers can also suffer from symptoms of postpartum depression.

A woman with PPD may feel like she has no maternal instinct and that she can't even take care of herself, let alone a baby. Worse yet, she may feel she has nowhere to turn.

Since I first spoke publicly about my journey through postpartum depression, I have received thousands of letters from women who are suffering to varying degrees with PPD. Some women described bouts of weeping, anxiety, and fatigue. Others endured mind-numbing dysfunction or thoughts of extreme behavior involving hurting themselves or their babies. One of the common threads in the letters was a plea for help in finding more answers, from which could come compassion, understanding, and insight into why women suffer from PPD. Some of the letters came from women who had been institutionalized and rejected by their families.

Is it any wonder PPD has been hidden away, hushed up, and ignored for so many years? After all, how do you find a way to explain to anyone, especially other women who see this as the most joyful time in your life, that you are in complete despair and emotional pain? How do you relate feelings of being cast into a wasteland void of familiarity? Where do you find the words to explain that you can hold a new life in your arms and still feel no hope for the future? Who will you tell that you're not sure you'll make it through this very day? How can you possibly talk about it when you know that it could result in people thinking you are selfish, irresponsible, or crazy, or, even worse, having your baby taken away from you?

These questions reflect the reason I wanted to write this book. As difficult as my experience with PPD was, I know that I was spared some of the severe symptoms that have caused women to lose their livelihoods and even their families.

I do understand, however, what it feels like to be searching for an answer, something to give you hope that you can and will be happy again. I've been there. I went through months when I was certain I would never feel like myself again, or even know who "myself" was. There were devastating days in the first couple of months following my son's birth that have stayed as near to my consciousness as if they had happened yesterday. It has been important to me to record these thoughts and feelings while they are still close to me, while I can still remember clearly what it feels like to struggle every day with PPD.

I am a very private person who has been in the public eye for thirty-eight of the forty-one years of my life. I know that all of us have our own issues and problems, things that we attempt to solve and find solutions to in our own ways. I've always felt that my problems were just that—mine. I have come to understand, however, that by choosing to make public this very private part of my life, I can call attention to the common plea of the women who have written to me and give one more voice to those who suffer with PPD. This book doesn't have all the answers. It does reflect something I believe is more important—that life is about the journey and how we react to each of our experiences. We can choose to let them stop us, or we can grow from them and move forward. I'm convinced that we are here to share our experiences so that no one has to pass through the dark times alone.

I truly feel women are the nucleus of life. We take care of our children, husbands, friends, neighbors, associates, schools, and communities. Women gracefully change the face of the world every day. We need to take care of one another. We have to nurture and support one another. We must share our knowledge.

What I have to offer is my very personal story. Why? Because, as you'll read in this book, in my most desperate hour a woman I care deeply about told me her personal story. Her words saved my life. I can also share information and the treatment methods that worked best for me, which I found in the conscientious hands of my doctor, Judith Moore. I've asked her to share some of her knowledge and healing methods in this book.

My story also contains some humor. I share some of the lighter moments of my life because humor has always kept me moving forward. One of my favorite sayings is "Tragedy plus time equals humor." (I guess if you're going to laugh about it in the future, you might as well laugh about it now.) Medical and natural sciences may be the foundations for healing, but for me the door to health has always been laughter. I've noticed that laughter shakes the tension from my neck and causes me to breathe deeper. The very funny comedian Louie Anderson once told me, "When you're laughing it's impossible to think about anything else." Perhaps it's those moments when we aren't worried and full of self-doubt and self-criticism that we can remember our original purpose: to live with joy. It is then that we can heal.

During my first appearance on *Oprah* (October 1999), I met and talked with a woman in the audience who was struggling with PPD. The pain in her eyes was as familiar as my reflection in the mirror. Her eyes remain vivid in my memory. It may be the same pain I would see in your eyes. If it is, and you are a woman with PPD, you are in my heart. Even if you feel you are at your lowest point, know that my heart is filled with hope and the belief that you can and will overcome PPD. Sharing my own experience will be worthwhile if this book helps you to feel less alone and gives you enough faith to hang on for a better day. Trust me, it will come. Take comfort right now in knowing that being a mother matters to you. You wouldn't be in this much pain if it didn't.

We need to pull open the curtain of silence and talk about the physical and emotional changes that happen during postpartum depression. We have not done others or ourselves any favors by pretending that these changes don't exist. Our daughters, who may be having children in the future, must be better prepared to recognize the signs of PPD, know what they need to do to take care of themselves, and not compromise those needs. I would never want any of my daughters to feel as alone as I did in my experience with postpartum depression.

Our sons will also benefit from our willingness to be honest about what it means to be female. By being open about our lives, we can help them to know a woman as a complete, multilevel person. They will understand that a woman is different from a man, emotionally as well as physically, and grow to value those differences.

As I celebrate my baby's first birthday, I also mark my own new course in life. I now know that we don't have to wait for the pain to get so bad that we just black out. I believe the first step is removing the mystery and the shame that comes with believing we are each alone in our experience.

MARIE OSMOND   *May 2001*

1

Behind the Smile

From this angle, you can see right up my skirt.

I learned at an early age how a young woman protects her image. If she's "sitting like a lady," no one can see up her skirt.

I'm not "sitting like a lady" now. I'm collapsed in a pile of shoes on my closet floor. Around and above me hangs my clothing, which is all I can see as I lean against the back wall of the closet. I can see straight up one of my skirts on a hanger right over my head. It looks like a long, dark tunnel with the exit sealed off. It looks like my life right now.

The skirt goes with one of my favorite suits. I've worn it to several happy occasions. I can recall the events, but I have no memory of what it feels like to be happy.

I sit with my knees pulled up to my chest. I barely move. It's not that I want to be still. I am numb. I can tell I'm crying, but it's not like tears I've shed before. My eyes feel as though they have moved deep into the back of my head. There is only hollow space in front of them. Dark, hollow space. I am as empty as the clothing hanging above me. Despite my outward appearance, I feel like a lifeless form.

I can hear the breathing of my sleeping newborn son in his bassinet next to the bed. My ten-year-old daughter, Rachael, opens the bedroom door and whispers, "Mom?" into the room, trying not to wake the baby. Not seeing me, she leaves. She doesn't even consider looking in the closet on the floor. Her mother would never be there.

She's right. This person sitting on the closet floor is nothing like her mother. I can't believe I'm here myself. I'm convinced that I'm losing my mind. This is not me.

I feel like I'm playing hide-and-seek from my own life, except that I just want to hide and never be found. I want to escape my body. I don't recognize it anymore. I have lost any resemblance to my former self. I can't laugh, enjoy food, sleep, concentrate on work, or even carry on a conversation. I don't know how to go on feeling like this: the emptiness, the endless loneliness. Who am I? I can't go on.

But I do. I have a house full of people who depend on me. I have a baby to take care of, children who need me, a husband, friends, and family who all expect me to get back to my regular life and obligations.

Somehow, I find myself standing up again. I pull something out of the closet to wear. I run a washcloth under the cold-water faucet and press it to my face. I manage mascara and some lipstick. My mother always said, "No matter what, always put on lipstick." I do. I change the baby and wrap him in a blanket. I feel exhausted just doing these simple things.

I go downstairs to my world, which feels like a prison. My oldest son, Stephen, is shooting baskets in the driveway with his cousin. My eight-year-old, Michael, has a new piece of artwork he wants me to tape on my bedroom door, next to the fourteen other drawings. My one-year-old daughter, Brianna, grabs me enthusiastically around the knees. There is a woman standing in the living room. Rachael introduces her as our new next-door neighbor who has stopped over with a plate of goodies as a welcome gift. I have fifteen messages on the answering machine saying, "Congratulations on the new baby," "When can you come to the office?" "Can we set up a photo shoot?" There is a pile of bills, business mail, and FedEx packages waiting for my attention on the dining room table. My two-year-old knocks over a basket of laundry, and it rolls down the stairs. The baby cries. He wants to be fed.

That's when the "Marie Osmond" persona kicks in. I smile. I was trained in my entertainment upbringing to smile constantly when I'm around other people, and now it's as natural to me as breathing. Rule number one: I am here to make sure that everyone else is happy. It's my job.

I smile at my little artist. I smile at my new neighbor and my daughter. I smile at my toddler. I smile about the phone calls, the overflowing mail, and the laundry scattered on the steps. I lift the baby over my shoulder, pat his back, and I smile.

My smile stays on my face even though my eyes feel like they sink farther back in my head. My body aches from my forehead to my feet. It is sabotaged with fatigue. My throat tightens to choke off unwanted emotions. I have no idea what to do next. I am a stranger in my own life. But I'm still smiling, which lets everyone know that I'm fine. "Marie Osmond" is always "fine."

No one guesses the truth. They can't see that I'm in a constant spiral, spinning into gloom. I feel it's inevitable that I will hit bottom. I thought I had been there before, but this feels so much lower. Right now, all my thoughts and feelings are locked away. I wish I could toss away the key and it would all be over. But it's not so easy. My smile is like a two-way mirror. I can see out, but no one can see in. No one sees what is going on behind the smile.

◆

The Osmonds began performing as a family in the early 1960s, years before my brother Donny and I were even school age. My father managed my four older brothers, Alan, Wayne, Merrill, and Jay, who toured as a singing quartet. This often left my mother home alone with Virl and Tom, my two oldest brothers, who are hearing impaired, Donny and me, who were preschoolers, and baby Jimmy.

At that time there were advertisements for a product called Compoz. Appropriately named, it was a pill marketed to frazzled homemakers and mothers. I don't know what the main ingredient was, but the commercials were catchy enough to make any woman looking for a little peace of mind want to rush off to the drugstore and stockpile it.

Donny and I were rambunctious playmates who never gave our mother a moment of rest. We couldn't possibly sit quietly with a book or a board game. We never spent an hour together without devising a major plan of action. It wasn't fun or worth our time unless there was physical activity involving digging, stringing something up, flooding, capsizing, leaping, leveling, or capturing. If we were awake, then something was always shaking and moving. My poor mother had to deal with our energy and imaginations. She'd find her shoes full of peanut butter, her best blankets being used as pirate ships in the mud, and her necklaces and bracelets buried in the yard as the pirate "loot." Unfortunately, we once lost the loot when our marker blew away, and the family spent the entire day digging up a freshly tilled half acre of land looking for Mother's jewelry box. Captain Marie and First Mate Donny didn't have imaginary parrots sitting on our shoulders anymore. We had our very real father breathing down our necks.

You've heard the expression "What goes around, comes around," and it sure came back around for me with my own two toddlers, Brandon and Brianna, who are only a year apart in age. I call them Pete and RePete. They are pressed from the exact same mold Donny and I were. Brandon is full of energy and daring feats, and Brianna is outspoken and can slyly maneuver her brother to do anything she wants. Hmm . . . I wonder where she learned that technique? My mother offers no suggestions. She just smiles. I'm pretty sure she's enjoying the payback. (By the way, Mother, remember the fire that started in the field next to our house that hot summer day? It wasn't the heat.)

One afternoon, when I was three and Donny was five, my mother left us unattended, for what I'm sure was only a total of three minutes, to step outside to the clothesline and take down the six dozen pairs of socks and three loads of T-shirts we went through every week. I don't remember the crime Donny and I committed that particular day; I just remember her being very angry when she came to check on us, so it must have been a household felony. We probably did some type of structural damage to the house. Believe me, the two of us could compete with any natural disaster.

Donny and I knew we would be in trouble, so we hid by crawling up on the stools under the kitchen table. We lay silently across two or three stools, holding our breath, hoping not to be found. I remember watching my mother's legs walk into the kitchen and hearing her raised voice: "Donny! Marie! Where are you?" My mother tells me all she heard was my tiny three-year-old voice coming from under the kitchen table as I whispered to Donny, "She needs some Compoz."

She laughs about it now, but I wonder how often she felt overwhelmed by all of her responsibilities. Did she ever take time for herself, or did her role as "Mother" absorb every minute of her life? It was a badge of honor then for a woman to remain composed, like the name of the product, in any situation. Few women would actually speak of the difficulties of being a female or a mother. Perfection for women in the sixties was a wrinkle-free skirt and blouse, a string of June Cleaver pearls, hair styled and sprayed not to move, high heels, a spotless home, clean-cut kids with good manners, and a happy, well-fed husband.

My mother was surrounded by men and boys. She never talked about what she went through as a woman, either physically or emotionally. I'm sure no one ever asked. She always appeared to be "fine." Hmm . . . I wonder where I learned that technique?

I'm in awe when I think about her life—giving birth to and raising nine children. (My mother washed cloth diapers for over twenty years!) I always saw my parents as two pillars holding up the family as well as the business. My mother was a complete partner with my father in holding the reins on their team of children. They helped to teach us to have a belief in God and encouraged us to seek out answers to our questions about religion. As a young girl, I had read the fundamentals of many religions and chose my belief, not because it was my parents' religion, but because it answered my questions. It has always been a source of strength and comfort for me. My parents guided each of us with intelligence, discipline, and devoted love safely into our adult years. My mother has always been my role model, and I believe my survival in the entertainment business is in large part due to my desire to be a strong woman like my mother. She is my hero.

I can vividly recall what it felt like to be alone and in a crumpled heap on the closet floor. I remember thinking that my mother would never have fallen apart like that. I was sure no one would understand what I was going through. I could have managed the pain. It was the shame that was destroying me.

2

Overnight Sensation

Entertainers who are described as "overnight sensations" have one thing in common: Their success was anywhere between five and twenty-five years in the making. They become the current sensation because they were able to take a talent and refine it into a craft with years and years of practice. In "Something Good," a song from *The Sound of Music*, the character Maria sings, "Nothing comes from nothing. Nothing ever could." I believe this applies to almost everything we go through day to day, both good and bad. It all comes from something. Every thought, habit, belief, and choice is the result of everything that has gone before. I have come to realize that how you face the moment at hand, whether it's good news, bad news, a situation out of control, or, in my case, postpartum depression (which ended up being all of the above), is determined by the accumulation of the countless "somethings" that make up your past. An overnight sensation, something that gets our attention by arriving fully formed from out of nowhere, is pretty rare.

My postpartum depression was "sensational" for me because I sensed it in every area of my life. It wasn't
"overnight," however. The normal hormonal changes I experienced, as most women do, after giving birth tipped the
apple cart for me, but the depression that resulted had been
in the making for years. My PPD wasn't the result of a onetime physical imbalance. Once the debilitating physical
symptoms of it were under control with the help of the
treatments Dr. Judith Moore describes later in this book, to
fully recover I found I had to look at my complete state of
being, not just physical, but every aspect.

I tell my children about the balance of our human elements: physical, social, mental, and spiritual, by comparing
it to the four legs of a chair. One of the legs on your chair can
become weak and break, and, chances are, you will still be
able to keep yourself upright by balancing your weight over
the other three legs. But if one leg breaks and the other legs
of the chair are so weak they just give way, you will find
yourself on the floor. I fell so hard it was clear that the legs
of my chair had been crumbling beneath me for years. I just
didn't know it. (Hey, Orkin man, I think I've got a little
termite problem!) The breaking of the "physical" leg only
exposed the weakness in other parts of my life.

Recently, I talked with a woman who feels she has lived
with postpartum depression for two years. She received help
to balance her hormones shortly after the depression began,
but the feelings of despair did not lift. She realized that she
would have to work at fixing the other areas of her life, the
other legs of her chair, if she was ever going to heal fully. But
she was afraid. She knew she would have to look deeply into
everything she had tried to hide, dismiss, or push away because it was too painful to acknowledge.

I too was hesitant to acknowledge that I had problems.
Like many women I know, I thought I could handle, by my-

self, whatever happened in one way or another. After all, women are caretakers by nature. We know how to fix things. I didn't need help . . . I was the one who gave help. It took the loss of what I consider to be one of the most important parts of my existence, giving, to finally admit that I was not fixing this problem.

For me, life feels purposeless if I can't be of service to other human beings. I have the strongest sense of myself when I am interacting with others and when I can help someone else to enjoy life more. Our whole world seems to work this way. The economic system is built on supply and demand. One produces what the other needs to live fully, down to the most basic needs. Even our ecosystem demonstrates this: the rain feeds the earth, the earth the trees, the trees the air. Crisis only occurs when the demand outweighs the supply.

My children were the reason I knew my life was in crisis. My last valuable resource, being able to give, was completely depleted. In my most devastating moments of postpartum depression, I found I had nothing left to give to the ones who needed me the most. I had to stop and save myself.

It wasn't simple. Sunk deep in depression, I found when I tried to throw myself a lifeline that I didn't have a self or even a life I could identify as my own. I was an accumulation of "somethings" that were no longer working for me: ideas, thoughts, and habits that I had absorbed and allowed to develop through past experiences. I had to ask if it was worth it to me to find myself. And where did I start?

The biblical commandment says to "love thy neighbor as thy self." It doesn't say to "love thy neighbor more than thyself." This comes from the Ten Commandments, not the Ten Suggestions. You can't give love or be of help to anyone else unless you have a self to use as a source. I couldn't ignore that it says to love oneself, either. I knew I would have to separate from the things in my past that were fueling the depression and find a way to love myself enough to be able to claim, "This is my life and I need to take care of it."

Until recently, I couldn't even fathom the courage it would take for me to say those words and mean it. First, according to my personal belief system, it felt like it was a selfish statement . . . as if I were only concerned with myself. Second, and perhaps even more frightening, it would mean that I was responsible for everything that had happened or would happen in my life, the past, the present, and especially the future choices I would make.

To get out of PPD, I first had to look at how I got into it. Few of us have histories that were intended to be harmful to us. (Though I do personally know people who grew up in horrendous situations. I am not discounting that reality.) But for all of us, what we absorbed through our daily environment played a part in the development of our selves.

It's not my intention to complain about my past. It was filled with great experiences and close and loving bonds with my parents and my brothers. I've never been a person who felt the need to talk about my hardships because no one's life, despite outward appearances, is problem free. But I've been told many times that I am perceived as having had a picture-perfect life. I guess it was assumed that if I had a problem, someone would take care of it for me, rescue me, or at the very least pay my way out of it. I believe it's pointless to speak of problems unless it's to make people aware of an issue that needs attention. I want to give some of my background because I believe it is part of what made me a candidate for postpartum depression. Though I certainly grew up under a unique set of circumstances, I don't believe the scenario will feel foreign to other women with postpartum depression. I have often felt that the stories women who have gone through depression have shared with me parallel my own upbringing and young adult life in many ways.

◆

My father and mother directed their household and our performing group using a one-for-all principle. It was how they chose to keep order in our lives with nine children, seven of whom had performing careers. My parents discouraged any one of us from complaining, and we were expected to always find the positive in our lives. There was no time or room for selfishness because it took every person to get the next show ready to go on.

In my young childhood years we would perform in one city, then break down our stage equipment, load the bus, and drive through the night to the next stop on the tour, trying to sleep curled up in a seat. In the new city we would unload the bus, launder our costumes, grab a shower, get a meal, do a sound check, rehearse, get into costume and makeup, do an hour of interviews and photos for the local press, and then go out on stage to perform again. (This was after we made it to the big time. Before this, we would perform three shows a day in three different towns.) Any spare time was spent answering fan mail and learning new songs. Before I began performing with my brothers, I would help my mother with the stage wardrobe and the packing. Then we would work the box office, counting the unsold seats and filling out the statements after every show. As soon as the show ended, the whole process started over again.

My parents raised us to believe that every family member was a key player in the success of our group and our family. I have deep respect for their determination that we each keep a clear perspective on the importance of the family as a whole instead of individual stars. It was understood that no solo success was possible without the efforts of the whole group, especially the original Osmond Brothers: Alan, Wayne, Merrill, and Jay. All earnings, whether from solo performances or from the entire group, were combined, as they would be in most businesses.

We were taught as children that our problems paled in comparison to those of many other people, including our two older brothers, Virl and Tom, who faced the difficulties of being hearing impaired. My parents felt that our fans and those who supported us paid hard-earned money to be entertained and it was our job to ensure that they left the show feeling that they'd had a great time. With this in mind, the only possible response to the question "How are you?" asked by anyone, at any time, was to smile and say: "Fine. Great."

I think I took this lesson a little too much to heart. In fact, I was consumed by the idea of never letting anyone see me as anything but happy, and it became an ingrained part of my personality. I became an expert at pushing my problems or needs out of my mind in order to deal with the day at hand and accomplish what needed to be done.

When I look back on this time in my life, I see myself as a little girl who had no time to just be a child. Though my parents put great effort into making sure our lives were as normal as possible by playing with us and sharing fun times, the fact still remains, our lives differed from those of most other children because we went to work almost every day. When other children were out playing, I was memorizing scripts, learning to sing a song in Swedish or Japanese for a foreign tour, and spending long days dancing, playing instruments, singing, and otherwise learning my craft. As hard as this may be to believe today, I was a shy, analytical little girl. I would first observe, and then listen to and measure everything people were saying or doing around me. I would study the way I looked in the mirror, and compare myself to my brothers. They were all thin and graceful, with thick, wavy hair and curly black eyelashes. I could barely find my eyelashes, my hair was straight and stringy, and let's just say that I had a tummy that always made an entrance before I did. It was just baby chubbiness, but it was a great source of humiliation for me and my feelings were rarely spared when it came to teasing.

Producers and directors bombarded me from all sides with "helpful" directions and criticism: "Walk this way, smile as you sing, dance this way, answer questions with these words." I was wearing fake eyelashes and a girdle by age eleven, just to try to look like I belonged in the family. If I had an idea or a way to express my individuality I was told "No." I became so used to this that I started telling myself no. "No, I don't have time for you." "No, you don't know anything." "Just be quiet and learn what they want." It didn't take me long to completely shut myself down so I could focus on what other people expected of me. Having aspirations of my own was equal in my mind to being selfish, and I didn't want that.

Many women have told me they received the same message while growing up. It was reinforced in their lives by praise or what they felt was acceptance. In my life, the normally positive quality of putting others first resulted in long-term negative effects because it was out of balance. Being professionally considerate to those who worked with me and to our fans was appropriate, but in some situations the consideration was not always returned in kind. The most hurtful result of this was that during my childhood and teen years, it sometimes took the form of abuse. I have never spoken about this publicly, and I would not consider doing so if I didn't feel it had significance in my battle with PPD. It wasn't until I began to heal from PPD, and I still consider myself to be in the process of doing that, that I completely understood the influence abuse had on me. Those experiences established in me a false perception that I had no right to personal boundaries. The levels of abuse varied from mild cases of blind ignorance to invasions of privacy.

In some situations I was treated more as a product than a person. This can be common in the entertainment business because it's your projected image, how the buying public recognizes you, that sells. In one instance when I was eleven, I was shooting a commercial for a Japanese soft drink. I had to sit in a boat, bouncing on the waves in the blazing heat every day for an entire week. One morning the boat overturned and we had to cling to the side of it in shark-inhabited waters until the crew came to the rescue. I was petrified by the time I got safely aboard, and my clothing and hair were wet and crusted with salt, but I was still required to stay out on the water. By late afternoon I was becoming seriously dehydrated. The sun beating down caused a burn on my legs that was so severe my skin later blistered, which made every step I took for the next week agonizing. Though there were supposedly child-care guardians present at the shoot, the bottom line was that everyone had been hired to get a commercial made, and that meant I was expected to get through it. My father became concerned about why we had not returned at the scheduled time. When he arrived at the location and saw what had transpired, he called for an abrupt end to it.

Mistreatment can come in many forms. It doesn't have to be severe. It can take the form of less intense, even excusable incidents that, repeated over time, have a long-term effect. For example, I spent many hours of my childhood in the recording studio. The producers, along with the studio band, would set the key in which the songs were recorded. I always tried to sing in the chosen key but often found that it was set too high for my voice. When I brought this to their attention, I was told that the key worked and sounded better for the musicians and the instrumentation, and it would not be changed. I would have to change. I would have to find a way to make it work. And that's exactly what I did. I would compromise my personal artistic standards because I didn't want to be a complainer or the one who held up a project. Over time, I grew to believe and accept that my input was the least important of all those involved in almost every project. This perception lasted well into my adult career.

Unfortunately, being unable to object in professional situations made me a candidate for the types of abuse that are intentional: being threatened, having my personal property intruded on or stolen, and, most damaging, being abused sexually.

I have spent many prayerful hours contemplating whether or not to reveal this part of my history. I found that my personal answer was that I can't be truthful about my experience with PPD without being honest about all the contributing factors. I have kept this private for a long time and will, for the most part, continue to do so because I truly believe it's pointless to discuss any particular incident. I refuse to make this be about the who, what, and where. I only want to make other women aware of how this part of my past, of which I had considered the effects to be long over, had significant influence on the severity of my postpartum depression. I feel it is an important part of the healing process for all women with PPD to look at what might be contributing factors for them.

I want to state that each incident was perpetrated by people who had very temporary access to my life. They were not people I have ever had a close relationship with, including my family, my friends, and business associates who have established careers working with me.

I also want there to be clarity about how this could happen. I was a protected child, well taken care of and guarded in every situation in which my parents believed there was any chance of danger. The abuse occurred in brief periods where it was assumed I was in a safe environment. My parents, and my brothers, were unaware of it until very recently, when I talked with them about my struggle with PPD and its effect on me. When they learned of this abuse, they expressed deep sadness and pain. They approached it from the perspective of "Where were we? Why didn't we know?" I explained that they couldn't possibly have known because I didn't communicate it to them. I was terrified to tell anyone what was happening because I was threatened, either for my personal safety or the safety and welfare of my family. When you are young you believe what you are told, and I believed these threats. I believed that revealing what was taking place would either endanger my brothers or parents or cause us to lose our livelihood because I had been told by the abusers that this is exactly what would occur. I thought they had the authority to make it true. Instinctively I knew the abuse was wrong, but I was unable to process and reason through the reality of it as an adult would, so I pushed it down and denied it.

As a parent, I know it's impossible to be with your child twenty-four hours a day. We can do everything possible to make sure they are in safe environments when we can't be with them, and then we have to trust that they have the resources to react appropriately if they sense danger. The awareness of abuse and the preparation for dealing with it have changed drastically in the last several years, but it was a hushed and shameful subject for previous generations.

Even today, the issue for me is not about the details of what happened. Those diminish in importance compared to the debilitating effects sexual abuse has on the human spirit and even the ability to function on a day-to-day basis. We may choose to ignore or hide abuse, but that doesn't mean it doesn't exist.

Appearances can successfully disguise reality. I was thinking recently about the time I spent growing up on farms. Many farms have what is called a manure pit, which is a large hole dug for the purpose of containing and disposing of everything that gets shoveled out of stables and barnyards. When it's full, the top becomes crusted over with soil, and often an incredible array of flowers will fill in and bloom, giving it the appearance of being a beautiful field. It's so convincing that you want to venture in to pick flowers, but take three steps and you'll find yourself knee-deep in all the unpleasant stuff buried underneath. Now that I'm speaking with women who are suffering or have suffered with PPD, I'm finding that emotional as well as sexual abuse is common in their pasts. We may have found beautiful ways to cover this, but something like PPD can break through the surface and expose those things we'd rather leave buried.

I thought in my case that I had dealt with the effects the abuse had on me. I had forgiven and found peace and left it in the past. What I didn't realize until I went for help with my postpartum depression was that I had never forgiven myself. Some part of me still felt that I was responsible. Because my right to maintain my personal boundaries during childhood had been abused and I had been unable to stop it, I thought I must have been doing something to cause it. I've since learned that this is a common perception among those with histories of abuse. As a child, you don't understand that being wronged doesn't mean you've done something wrong. I spread that feeling of responsibility over everything else that happened well into my adult life. I looked at it all in a self-critical way: What had I done wrong to deserve this? Was it my fault? I must have done something to bring on this pain. This, I think, is why, at age thirty-nine, taken over by PPD, I still thought: "What did I do wrong? I'm in pain. I deserve it. It's my fault." I had years and years of practice at self-blame. My boundaries as a person had been first invaded and then shattered. My sense of self had faded away slowly, and as time passed I lost faith in my ability to determine what was right for my own life. It was with this attitude that, as an adolescent, I was thrown into the national spotlight and forced to find a way to survive with my life under inspection.

◆

W hen I was fourteen years old, Donny and I starred in our own television variety show, the Donny & Marie show. Though doing the show was an exciting and phenomenal experience for a teenager, being in the public eye had huge drawbacks for me. My days were usually eighteen hours long. For my education, I was tutored on the set a minimum of three hours a day. We had a new script to memorize every week, and at least five songs with choreography to learn for each show. There were ice-skating routines and comedy sketches to learn (though the word comedy is debatable if you look at the original shows). Many shows had up to twelve costume changes, which called for at least four hours of fittings every week. The studio made sure my hair, my nails, and my skin looked perfect every day because they also scheduled me for outside events and public appearances. Dates with boys were out of the question because I had no free time.

Donny and I were given the nickname One-Take Osmonds by the producers and the crew on the show. It was meant as a compliment on our professionalism. When it came time to tape the shows, the director and crew never had to stop rolling tape because of mistakes on our part. We would stay at rehearsals until the dance steps were perfected, the lines were memorized, the spins on the ice rink were up to Olympic standards, and the songs were recording-studio ready. If the words "take two" were heard on tape days, it meant that we had failed at our jobs, disappointed people, imposed on our guest stars, and wasted time and resources.

One-Take Osmond became the motto for my very existence. My self-worth was tied to my ability to do it all right the first time, thereby making everyone happy.

One afternoon during our first season, after an eight-hour rehearsal, I was heading off to a costume fitting with books and scripts in my arms and ice skates over my shoulder. One of the senior executives caught up with me in the parking lot. He had a disapproving look on his face. I thought I had been doing a good job, but I could see that my best wasn't good enough for him. He told me directly that unless I lost weight the show would be canceled. More than two hundred people would lose their jobs, and it would be on my conscience because I couldn't keep food out of my mouth. He didn't spare any words in telling me that I was an embarrassment to the show and to my family. He suggested, while wearing a glued-on grin, that I keep this conversation to myself. If I told any adults he said he would deny it. I was so humiliated I couldn't speak.

Not only did I feel responsible for contributing to the financial support and image of my own family, I felt the pressure of supporting more than two hundred other families. The message was driven home hard. At an age when most girls feel awkward about natural body changes anyway, my self-esteem was shattered. I was five feet, five inches tall and weighed 103 pounds, but on TV the image flattens, causing a person to look ten pounds heavier. For this reason, many women in television and film want to maintain their weight at least ten pounds below normal.

On the show, I was being compared at every turn with adult females who were my peers in the business, women with refined looks and features and attitudes to match. I was expected, for the sake of my job, to be as sexy as Charlie's Angels, as cute and sassy as Olivia Newton-John, and as skinny as Cheryl Tiegs. Here I was, a girl going through puberty, trying to pull off an adult life, trying to measure up as I stood next to the most beautiful female stars of that time. Imagine being sixteen and trying to feel good about yourself while you're standing next to Raquel Welch. The studio would even send Donny and me to have our facial pores vacuumed out every so often because we couldn't even have a teenage pimple.

I made my best effort to live up to what was expected of me. I spent the next four years in a harmful cycle of fad diets, diuretics, brief bouts with purging, and starving myself to ninety-three pounds to create the image that was required for national television. One day, my wardrobe person came into the dressing room to report that a female guest star, a television beauty, was anxious about being on camera with me. She had overheard this star telling the producer that I was so pretty and thin that she knew she would look terrible next to me. I heard the word *thin* and felt overjoyed. I was ecstatic that someone saw me as thin; I felt I had finally succeeded. I sailed through the show that day, until during one of the costume changes while dressing into one of the ice-skating leotards, I caught a glimpse of my back in a trifold mirror. I remember staring at the protrusion of my bones from my shoulders all the way down my back. I was shocked at the stick-thin appearance of my legs and arms. It was no longer thrilling to be thin. To be honest, it looked life threatening. I had starved myself to the point of losing my muscle and skin tone, and it was ugly to my eye. My joyous reaction from earlier that day turned into fear at my own self-neglect. I had hidden it well under clothes, but it was obviously taking its toll.

The sad part is that then we just didn't know any better. Nutrition took second place to beauty for most women. Not much was said about the effects of dieting, and weight was taken off in any way that worked. Just look back at all the diet crazes that came and went during the seventies and eighties. We were a nation of girls and women determined to look like Twiggy no matter what.

At other times, I had to go to extreme measures just to make it through a show. During an ice-skating routine in the middle of taping a show, Donny accidentally skated over my finger. My fingertip swelled up to the size of a strawberry, and I could feel the painful throbbing all the way up my arm and into my head.

The network representatives and the producers held a quick meeting about what should be done. Stopping the taping would cost the show thousands of dollars in overtime because they would have to keep the crew on standby while I went to the hospital. They concluded that I would be required to finish the show and could be taken for medical attention as soon as it was over.

I knew there was no way I could resume the show because the pain was causing me to feel both nauseated and faint. After I heard the decision, I went backstage to the scene shop, where the carpenters build the sets, and found an electric drill. I rested my hand on a worktable, aimed the drill over my pulsing fingernail, closed my eyes and pushed the trigger. Blood spurted like a break in a water main. I sat down on the floor in tears until my favorite stage manager, Sandy Pruddin, found me. Seeing me there, pale and trembling, he lifted me in his arms and carried me to my dressing room. He was very angry about the decision to not take me to the hospital. Sandy worked on most of our shows including the talk show until the time of his death. He always treated me first as a person and then as an entertainer. He stepped in with directness and action if he thought anything that was happening during the shows would compromise my safety. He was an unforgettable person with great heart.

During another incident I took a fall from a platform eight feet above the stage. We had rehearsed a dance number the day before that included high kicks and quick steps. Overnight, the set was readied for the actual shows with fresh wax applied on the platforms and the stage. While taping the show, I was performing the dance number as rehearsed up on the platform, when I lost footing on the slippery surface and crashed to the floor below. I landed with a blow to the back of my neck, stunning the nerves leading to my arms and legs. I couldn't move. The executives and producers gathered around me, discussing what to do while encouraging me to try to sit up. Sandy pushed through the group, lifted me from the floor and carried me off the set. Complete feeling returned to my arms and legs about twenty minutes later. The feeling also came back to my neck with bone-wrenching pain, a permanent injury I still deal with to this day. Though I probably should have been taken to the hospital to be checked for bone and nerve damage, I felt incredible pressure to go back out and finish taping the show. Worse than the pain of either accident was the deep injury it caused to my self-worth. I felt I was a product that should be refurbished and back in working order as soon as possible.

I was accumulating years of thoughts, habits, and choices that had many long-term effects on my sense of well-being. I couldn't continually mistreat my body to look good on the outside and not suffer the consequences on the inside, though at that time I couldn't see an alternative.

My body began to pay up in full once the show was off the air and I had met and married my first husband. I was so elated at the prospect of establishing a home and starting a family. I had always seen children as a big part of my life.

Pregnancy, as it turns out, was not as easy for me as for my mother, who had given birth every two years from the first child to me. Jimmy is three years younger. One of the reasons may have been the result of a severe hereditary potassium deficiency doctors discovered in my teenage years. Other women in my family had dealt with the same problem, but mine was complicated by the fact that my kidneys were functioning at a reduced rate. The trauma my body had gone through nutritionally during adolescence may have also contributed. Your body knows when it has weaknesses and protects you from stressing it further.

So I was out-of-my-head thrilled when, at age twenty-three, I carried my first baby. I was also out-of-proportion huge! I gained sixty-five pounds during the pregnancy. It was more important to me that my baby have nutrition than that I maintain an image, so I ate. I think my undernourished cells formed a pact to grab any nutrients they could and store them for the future and even eternity. I'm sure I was rebelling against watching every bite I took. Pregnancy was the best excuse to finally fill up.

Following the dissolution of my first marriage, before my son, Stephen, was even two years old, I struggled daily with my self-esteem. My every thought held anger toward myself. I felt I didn't add up. I wasn't good enough. I could never be pretty enough, and once again I wasn't thin enough. These were not the reasons my marriage had ended, but they were residual feelings that stayed with me for years.

◆

It took me a long time to open up to the possibility that someone could be attracted to me for who I was both inside and out. But then I met Brian Blosil. He was funny and charming. His priorities were very similar to mine: a strong relationship to God, a dedication to his family, and a love for children. He also had great clarity when it came to drawing the line between what was right and wrong for him. He helped me learn how to recover and set my own boundaries. Actually, he was so careful about not imposing on me that I had to ask him to marry me. I married Brian, and in fourteen years together we have been blessed with six children.

Brian is also from a large family; he is the oldest of seven children. His mother, Georgia, and I talked recently about what it's like to raise a large family in the new millennium as opposed to the sixties, when she had young children. She remembered how excited she felt the day she had her first washer and dryer delivered and hooked up in her house.

She said that when her mother came for a visit, she pointed out that now instead of doing the laundry just once a week, Georgia was doing a couple of loads every day. She told Georgia: "You've caused yourself more work. Before, the kids wore their overalls for more than one day and you used a bath towel three or four times. Now you're washing them every day."

Georgia confirmed the accuracy of her mother's words. It seemed the laundry never let up. She also felt she became isolated in a way she didn't expect. Before the home washer and dryer, a woman could meet up with other women to share the once-a-week laundry duties, which gave them time to socialize, talk through common problems, and feel a sense of camaraderie. I think it was like a cheap form of therapy that was mutually beneficial.

We are meant to be social beings. We feel the need to be in a group, to surround ourselves with others who experience life in a similar way. Raising children is a monumental daily commitment, and it's easy to constantly question if you are making good decisions, both large and small. For young mothers to be in contact with other women provides a comfort zone where they can safely share their concerns as well as their joys.

With computers, online shopping and banking, home

delivery services, air-conditioning, and an appliance for whatever need you might have, there is almost no reason to leave the house anymore. We have become so self-contained that it's easy to fall into a pattern that doesn't include real communication or emotional support from others, especially other women facing the challenges of raising children.

I isolated myself early in my postpartum depression because I was going through the same feelings of not adding up, that my best wasn't good enough. I'd also never known any women who had experienced emotions of such an extreme nature after childbirth, which left me feeling even more alone.

My children provided me with the courage to save myself. In actuality, they demanded it, as only kids can. Children have voices that cut through the confusion because they have an intuitive understanding of how to keep balance in their lives. If they need contact with others, they seek it out. When they're hungry, they find food. They weep when sad and laugh when something strikes them as funny. They protect what is important to them and share freely when they know the supply is ample. Where else but through the eyes of these little ones can we see clearly our own weaknesses, imperfections, selfishness, and impatience? They help us grow in character as they grow in stature. Observing my children helped me to rediscover my intuitive self. I had always trusted and used my intuition when it came to my children and my business life. Now I had to listen to it to know what I needed and how to take care of myself. I'm just now learning that it is possible to be a whole person each and every day and still have the ability to nurture, care for, and love others. Not because I feel they need it, but because I want to give it. It wasn't an "overnight sensation," but I have the second half of my life to practice.

3

I Know They're Mine

My kids are washing up in a bucket in the backyard. I could tell you that it's the only way I've found to keep the bathroom clean, but they're actually doing it for fun. It's "pioneer day" at the Blosils'.

Two or three times a year, Brian and I set aside a whole day and night to honor our ancestors: no television, no lights, no microwaves, no Nintendo or Walkmans or hair dryers. We even unplug the phones. (Yes, I still wear lipstick. I figure even the Native Americans had henna!) I'm pretty sure the kids would vote to have pioneer day once a week. They love for Brian and me to tell stories by candlelight as they sit in a circle around us, wrapped in blankets. They look forward to the challenge of making every meal over a barbecue and they are convinced that the pioneers invented the shish kebab.

I don't know if that's true, but I did tell them that pioneer children invented shoulder and foot massages because they knew their parents had to walk so far every day carrying heavy loads. It's amazing what you can get kids to do if they think it's a game. This one is usually good for forty minutes of pure bliss.

At least once a year we load up the car and take off to a place that is wild and free, a place remote and unknown . . . like a state park with the kind of campgrounds that feature indoor hot showers every fifty yards. (Hey, I respect and appreciate nature. I just don't want to smell like it.)

We used to try to get by with only the bare necessities on these trips. I wanted my kids to really experience the world as God designed it, until one time that world threw a tantrum that made me question why I ever left the safety of our home.

We went camping for a weekend with some friends who had a deluxe motor home extraordinaire. This four-star hotel on wheels had everything except an address. Our friends invited us to share the comforts of their motor home with them, saying there was plenty of sleeping room for all. (That should tell you how big it is.) But no, I insisted we were in the wilderness to be as one with the earth and that we would be sleeping in our eight-man tent.

I zipped each of the kids into their sleeping bags and turned out the lantern. We lay quietly, listening to the sounds of the owls and the crickets . . . and our neighbors playing Nintendo and making popcorn in their microwave. It smelled delicious. In the middle of the night, I was awakened suddenly by the sounds of my older kids screaming and the little ones crying. It was pitch-black and there was a terrifying noise, like the *Wizard of Oz* flying monkey troops descending and trying to carry us off, tent and all, back to the witch's castle. I tried to sit up and went face first right into the roof of the tent, which was four inches above me. A freakish, almost hurricane-type wind had picked up during the night, bending our support poles to the ground and flattening the tent. Of course, it was hard enough to locate one another, let alone flashlights, and when a tent is collapsed, it's no pioneer picnic trying to find the entrance.

After the escape, we ended up tapping on our friends' motor home door at two in the morning. They waved us in and started pulling out blankets and pillows. It seemed that everything in this mammoth contraption could be converted into a bed. Don't ask me to explain. I think one of the kids slept on the mini–trash compactor, which folded out to become a bed. Before the microwave was turned into a sleeping surface, we warmed up pizza bagels and then fell back to sleep by the light of the television.

In today's world of satellite dishes and cell phones, it's easy to lose our resourcefulness, especially when it comes to survival basics. I'm just as guilty as the next person of indulging in the best that modern technology has to offer. I'm sure I'd be the record holder in the magnetic-strip dash. No one can whip a credit card out of her wallet and through a swipe machine faster than I can. It's a talent, developed over time by shopping for clothes with seven kids. Sometimes the card almost melts in my hand, moving from one hot buy to another.

I'd also be lost without my cell phone . . . literally. I have absolutely no sense of direction. I've been known to run to the grocery store in L.A. and end up crossing the border into Mexico. I'll call Brian, and if we're in Utah, he'll say something like: "See the big mountain range? That's east." I'll say: "I'm between the drive-through malt shop and the place where we bought the double stroller. Just tell me how to get home."

It's obvious I never would have made it as a pioneer woman. You can't chart a new course with no sense of direction. I can see myself wandering away at the first rest stop and being left behind. The pioneers ventured on a courageous journey, following only rough maps and their instincts in hopes of finding homelands where they could prosper and raise their children. Instead of Salt Lake City, I probably would have led the Mormons into Anchorage, Alaska, saying the whole time, "I know the snow's gonna let up any day now. Boy, this is one long night. How about a midnight snack?"

I am fascinated by the journal entries preserved from the pioneer days, especially those written by women. The necessary level of perseverance and sacrifice on their part is inconceivable in today's world. Talk about the bare necessities. These women had only whatever comfort nature provided, depending on their location. I'm pretty sure this didn't include a lighted makeup mirror. Their journal entries are full of hardships and sorrow, illness, and fear of attack. I bet that if these women had postpartum depression they never even felt the symptoms. My worst PPD day was probably like a holiday for these gals. The most intriguing entries are their recordings of deep, intuitive feelings about what their future would hold, from marriage to childbirth to their own fate.

My mother is an avid journal keeper, and taught each of us as children to write about our days. We wrote about events, our travels, and people we met on tour. It was one of her ways of helping us feel grounded no matter where we were geographically. I still try to write in mine every night about what happened throughout my day: the kids' accomplishments and funny things they do and say. I told my mother that it would be embarrassing to have someone else read my journals because almost every entry, from the day my first child was born to the present, ends with the same two words: "I'm exhausted." She laughed and said she had recently looked through her own journals and had had the same revelation. In all her years of raising nine children she almost always ended each entry with the same words.

One of my friends was showing me a journal written by an ancestor who, with her husband, was settling farm property in upstate New York in the early 1800s. As I turned each brittle page, she pointed out to me that almost every entry had the same two words: "I'm exhausted." I guess it's the universal language among women. I mean, it's lasted two hundred years!

Most of my journal entries aren't detailed. I usually only have the energy at night for one or two descriptive lines, and sometimes it's even impossible to read those because I'll doze off and leave a long pen-mark trail across the page and off the edge. Talk about your run-on sentence!

Scattered throughout my journals over the years are entries in which I've written a few lines about an intuitive feeling I've had. I rarely shared these feelings with anyone at the time because there was no logical basis for them, which made them difficult to explain. The entries that show the most foresight are those I wrote about the children I sensed would come into my life.

I've always been open about the fact that some of my children are adopted. Brian always felt that the number of children we had was an issue that should be left to me. He believed that God would provide and direct me concerning the size of our family, and he respected my judgment as the mother. When I was a little girl I always pictured myself with a large family. As an adult, I didn't give much thought to adoption because I was able to give birth to my first child. The idea of adopting came from a couple I'd known for a number of years who had an adopted child. They knew how much I wanted more children and told me they would be happy to talk with me about it. They gave me all the information about the process and said they would make a request to the agency they had used on my behalf if I felt this was something I wanted.

Following that conversation, Brian and I spent the rest of the day talking through the idea. I wanted more children with all my heart. I went to sleep that night still unsure about what to do.

There are times when an intuitive feeling can come over me so strongly that it's hard to ignore the message. The next day I told Brian I could sense a little child who seemed to be mine. I recorded this in my journal. I felt an incredible peace about putting our names on a list to adopt. He agreed that while we waited he would have time to find the peace that this was right for us as well. I had no doubt that it was. I left it in God's hands, and we went on with our lives.

Eventually, the day arrived when someone from the adoption agency called to say that a young woman had decided that her baby would be placed for adoption. She gave us the details of the situation and asked if we'd be interested. I didn't even have to pause for breath. Absolutely, I was interested. I was so excited, I wanted to see the baby right then, but the agency representative said that wasn't possible. My heart skipped a beat or two until I was told the baby was still months away from being born. I would have to wait patiently. Patience is not in the top three on the list of my good personal qualities. I'm not sure it's on the list at all. I've been known to eat dessert before dinner . . . more than once.

◆

One afternoon, a couple of weeks later, I was in a meeting with my agent at William Morris. We were going over my calendar for the next year when a phone call came through from Bob Hope. He wanted to know if I was available to join him for an upcoming USO tour in the Middle East. We would be traveling from ship to ship by helicopter to entertain the troops. Brian was at the meeting as well, and

I could see his eyes light up with interest. He's always ready for adventure. I had been on tour with Bob Hope before. The USO shows are always fun, and Bob is a great host. The troops are so responsive and appreciative that many entertainers jump at the chance to perform for them. Bob was ready to lock in a lineup of performers for this tour, and needed an answer immediately. I wasn't sure why, but I didn't feel right about going. I didn't want to disappoint Brian or Bob, but the uneasy sensation persisted through that day and night. The next day Brian revealed to me that he was also feeling hesitant. Meanwhile, Bob had gone out of his way to clear it with the military so we could bring our son, Stephen, who was only four, along with us. It seemed as though everything was perfectly in place, but I still had a strong feeling that I needed to stay home. I declined the tour, which gave me feelings of regret at the thought of disappointing people, especially since I couldn't put my finger on the reason I wasn't going.

Two months later I got a message from my office that the adoption agency had called and I needed to contact them right away. I don't even know how I dialed the phone or what I said to the office assistant at the agency, but somehow she managed to decipher that it was me calling. (She was probably used to incoherent babbling . . . and I don't mean from the babies. I mean from the overexcited parents-to-be.) She calmed me down enough for me to listen to what she was saying.

"Your baby has been born," she told me. "There was a miscalculation on the due date. Can you come to pick her up in a couple days?"

Our little girl was here! I could have heard that news over and over again and never tired of it.

"Yes," I told her, and thanked her so profusely that she probably felt as if she were the one who had given birth. I ran to find Brian and we hugged and cried until we finally snapped back into reality about all we had to do to get ready. I was super commando: "Dry your eyes. We've got some shopping to do! Meet me in the car. Think pink and move it!"

Three days later we were in a hotel room near the hospital where the baby had been born, standing by for a call from the agency about what time to pick her up. My "waiting patiently" clock had run out, and I was a bundle of nerves. Brian tried to distract me by turning on the television. I was pacing the other side of the room when he called me over and said, "I can't believe this. Look at what's on right now." We watched on the news as Bob Hope and the USO performers turned to wave at the cameras and boarded a plane for the Middle East. We both stood there in awe, knowing that if we had been on a plane to leave the country, our baby girl might have gone to another name on the waiting list.

The call finally came to pick our baby up from the nursery. My heart was pounding as we were pointed to a little girl in a bassinet. As darling as this baby was, I felt instinctively that she wasn't supposed to be our daughter. I was very close to crying when a nurse approached me and said, "I'm so sorry. You were misdirected. Your little girl is over here."

And there she was—my gorgeous, treasured, angelic baby. The child I had sensed so strongly, the one I had described in my journal. My joy knew no limits. I was her mother and I knew she was my daughter.

I knew this wasn't mere coincidence, but that it was God's plan that this child should be with us. Following that first experience I began to pay closer attention to my intuitive feelings and record them in my journal. I have felt the presence of each of my children before they entered my life. I know this type of foresight is not unique to me. I've heard and read countless stories of women feeling the presence of their children in many situations. Whether it was sensing a child in trouble from afar, or being led to help or take in a child they didn't even know, they felt an unexplainable attachment to the child.

I was on the *Larry King Live* show in the spring of 2000, along with actresses Donna Mills, Nell Carter, and Valerie Harper. The topic was adoption. I thought it was fascinating that these women reported similar experiences to mine when it came to being a mother. They felt they knew their children had chosen to be with them, and each woman expressed certainty that they were connected with the exact child they were supposed to parent.

On *Donny & Marie,* we dedicated a whole hour to adoption. Two young birth mothers came on the show, along with one of the couples who had adopted one of their babies. In both cases, the birth mothers said they had chosen the adoptive parents from photographs in files of prospective parents. Each young woman had the same overwhelming feeling when looking at the photographs that she had found the parents of her baby. It was impossible not to be moved by the testimony of these young women and the conviction they felt about their babies' being with the right adoptive parents. One of the birth mothers told a story about thinking of a name for her baby right after the birth. She told no one about it. A week later, the adoptive mother called to tell her that they had decided to name their new daughter Lauren and wanted to know if she felt okay with the name. The birth mother took it as another sign that she had chosen the right parents because Lauren was the name she had picked. It wasn't the young women who were shedding tears during this show; they seemed assured they had made the right choice. It was the rest of us: audience, crew, executives, and producers, all weeping at this brief moment of witnessing the best that life has to offer . . . human beings in perfect communication with one another and with God.

The feelings I have for my adopted children are the same as those I have for the ones I carried. I am often asked by the media which of my seven children are adopted. I always reply, "I can't remember. There is no difference."

That is the truth. They're all mine. I didn't expect any of them, so every time another child came along, I was both surprised and grateful. When I had one child, I thought, "How great." With my second I thought, "Perfect, they can share growing up together." When the third child arrived, I felt incredibly blessed. It was more than I had dreamed possible. After the fourth baby, it felt like a perfect family, with six members. (And we could all still get in one car.) With my fifth baby, I remember thinking, "This is amazing. God must have a lot of faith in me." On the arrival of my sixth, I felt that "I'd better have a lot of faith in God." When I was having contractions with my seventh, I think I shouted, "By the way, didn't you tell us to cease our labors on the seventh?"

Having each of my children has been a blessing, a life-changing experience. I don't mean a onetime adjustment, I mean life-changing every day. I cherish every twenty-four hours I have with them. That doesn't mean my life as a mother has been simple or easy. I don't think it is for any mother. It's not easy to guide a child through all the choices available in life, especially knowing that ultimately they will end up making their own choices. The umbilical cord does not function outside of the womb. How quickly independence takes hold. There's a reason for that. All mothers hold their breath when their little ones take a first unassisted journey down a flight of stairs, but that doesn't mean we can or even want to stop them from trying.

As joyful as motherhood can be, it has also proven, in my life, to hold moments of deep sorrow as well. I wasn't a stranger to depression in connection with my children before I went through PPD. A couple of years earlier, I suffered a form of despair without actually going through the birth process. It wasn't until after I appeared on *Oprah* to talk about PPD that I learned from her panel of experts that adoptive mothers, due to stress and the sudden change in their lives and schedules, can also suffer almost every symptom of postpartum depression.

◆

I was getting ready to play Anna in *The King and I* on Broadway. It was a fast rehearsal process because they wanted to have me take over the role as soon as I could. I was in a whirlwind, learning a British accent, memorizing the script, rehearsing the choreography and the music, getting my voice in shape, having costumes fitted (let me tell you, when they tighten that corset, it's no problem hitting the high notes). I also wanted to figure out ways to make the character unique for me. The kicker was that I had to be ready to go on stage in seventeen days. This was one of those times I had to put my faith in God that I would be able to accomplish it all. Following the opening, I was thrilled and grateful for the great reviews I received, especially when a *New York Times* critic noted that my British accent was so flawless you could drink tea and eat cucumber finger sandwiches with it. Faith does work wonders.

At the same time I was rehearsing *The King and I,* I was doing a holiday show in Atlantic City. I would perform two shows a night on the weekends in Atlantic City, then drive back to New York City for the Broadway rehearsals on the weekdays. To this day, I still mix up the two shows. Does the song "Shall We Dance?" have the words "one-horse open sleigh" in it?

We decided, as a family, to all be in New York City together while I was performing in *The King and I.* Besides my double performing duties, Brian and I needed to think about our housing and schools for the older children. I wanted to have the transition be as smooth as possible, knowing they were all moving to accommodate my work.

About six weeks prior to starting rehearsals, I had an intuitive feeling that there was a baby girl who was supposed to come to our family, and I felt that she would arrive by Christmastime. Later that week, I was feeling I should make a phone call to a specific friend to talk to her about these impressions. My friend actually laughed and reminded me that it was already October and there was no way to find and adopt a baby by Christmas. I told her that I had to act on my feelings and call. I knew from past experience that if it was supposed to happen, it would.

I put the thought aside and threw myself into getting prepared to play Anna. About seven days before we were set to relocate the family from Utah, I was alone in my hotel room in New York after rehearsal. I experienced the same strong feeling about the baby girl. That night I got on my knees and prayed. When I looked at how busy my life was, it seemed impossible to take on another child, especially considering that my youngest at that time was just turning one. If it was going to happen, there was a very small window of opportunity. It needed to take place in the next four days, before I opened on Broadway. Once I was performing full-time, it would be impossible to leave New York.

The next morning there was a voice mail message from the friend I had called in October. In the background I could hear the cooing sounds of a newborn as my friend said, "You will not believe what has happened. This is a miracle. Your baby girl flew in with the stork. Call me."

I burst into tears and called Brian, who was at home in Utah with the children. At first he was terrified that something had happened to me because I could hardly put words together. I was finally able to stop crying long enough to say, "She's here. You have to go get her right now."

Brian had to really scramble to get an infant car seat,

baby formula, nursing bottles, and an adorable pink layette especially for the new baby. He then drove to pick her up and bring her home. The next night, I was able to catch a flight home to take my new daughter in my arms. It was as miraculous to me as if she had come from my own body, and I knew it was perfect unity between a child and her family.

What I'd love to write next is that we all went off to New York and lived happily ever after, but that's a fairy tale . . . and this was Broadway.

◆

Under the best of circumstances, starring in a Broadway show can be physically grueling and emotionally draining. I can understand how it doesn't appear that way because it looks like so much fun, and it really is, but it's also intense, concentrated effort. It's difficult to describe the output of energy demanded on stage during those three and a half hours, but I can probably come close by comparing it to being the host of a large party at your house. You've picked out a new outfit, done your hair and makeup, called everyone on your guest list, shopped, planned, and prepared all day. The guests arrive hungry and expecting to be entertained. You know it's important to have a chance to talk to everyone individually, but at the same time you have to make sure the whole party is running smoothly. Everyone is looking to you for direction, and you are responsible for making sure your guests are enjoying themselves. You know how at the end of a party you've hosted, you feel so happy but completely exhausted from sucking in your stomach all night? Now imagine throwing that party eight times a week. It's kind of like that. You also need to keep up your stamina, take care of yourself so you don't get sick, and not talk much during the day so your singing voice is strong for the show. On your day off, traveling to places where you could possibly get stuck is out of the question. As they say, "The show must go on!" and it can't if you aren't doing your part. But I wouldn't trade performing a single show, because I love it. It's hands down one of the best jobs I can think of.

My family and I lived in a hotel through the holidays, after which we planned to move to a brownstone in Manhattan. We were for the most part existing out of suitcases, which was challenging with a newborn baby and my one-year-old son, Brandon. The laundry alone was killer. My other kids are such road warriors from traveling and touring with me that they set up camp in a hurry and seemed content getting caught up in the excitement of New York City at Christmastime.

Mornings were set aside to spend time with the kids and finalize the plans for the town house and schools. I also wanted to be with the newborn as much as I could. We hired babysitters so the older kids would be able to go out on their own activities. Press interviews and photo sessions for *The King and I* took up several mornings a week early in the run. The holidays were fast approaching, and Brian and I were planning ways to make Christmas special and fun for the kids even though we would be spending it in a hotel room. Before I went to the theater at night, I would get dinner for the kids. Notice I said "get" and not "make." This meant, on most nights, opening the door, paying the delivery person, and getting out the paper plates. I would hop in a car to get to work by six o'clock for makeup and vocal warm-ups. On Wednesdays and Saturdays I would have to be at the theater by noon because we did two shows, a matinee and an evening performance. The rest of life was so hectic that for the most part I found being on stage relaxing. At least the order of events was scripted and I knew what was going to happen next, unlike in our lives.

By Christmas Eve, I was exhausted from weeks of getting up several times during the night to feed the baby and anxious because I didn't have everything prepared for Christmas Day. I left Brian with a list of last-minute gifts and grocery needs and went to do the show. Following the first act I came off stage to find Brian waiting for me in the wings. I asked him if he had been able to get everything on the list and he said no. I was so tired that I got instantly upset and said, "How are we supposed to finish the shopping? The stores are closed for the night. The things on that list were important for Christmas."

It only takes a brief moment to rearrange your priorities. Any thoughts of Christmas left my head in the moment Brian took my arm and said, "Marie, something's happened. There's been an accident."

There is no news more frightening than those words. I've been the recipient of my share of bad news, from business problems to illnesses, but nothing compares to being a mother and hearing the word *accident*. You feel an incredible and unbearable panic. Your child is in danger and you are helpless to stop it. Your reality goes into slow motion. You want to shift it into reverse, but the gears are locked and you're forced to face the disaster ahead.

Brian followed me to my dressing room, where he explained that Brandon had been taken to the emergency room with third-degree burns on his ankle, foot, and both of his hands. With everyone so crowded in the hotel, the nanny had briefly set the bottle sterilizer on the floor to make room on the counter to fix snacks for the kids. It only took that one minute for my one-year-old to crawl over and tip it toward himself, splashing the boiling water on his hands and down his leg to his foot.

One vivid memory of that time remains, the one of my small child in a hotel crib with his foot, leg, and hands wrapped in gauze. He wasn't crying, but the expression in his eyes broke my heart in a million pieces. His sweet little eyes searched my face as if to say, "Mommy, what's going on? What happened to me?"

The doctors gave us instructions on how to change our son's bandages three times a day. They told us we would have to wait for a couple weeks, through the initial healing process, to see if his foot would require skin grafts.

All I could think was, "This is too much for me; I don't know if I can take it." I know I went into a state of shock at first and then, in the days that followed, a silent type of depression.

Every time I held Brandon, or changed the bandage, I was filled with heart-wrenching regret. The nanny who had been there that night is one of the most loving, dedicated people I could possibly find to help me with my children. She was devastated, but I knew that it had been an accident, and the truth is, we are all capable of being involved in one at any time.

Having to leave my kids to go to work every day became almost more than I could stand. My older children were upset because I was so distraught about their brother's injury. I craved time to bond with the new baby, take care of Brandon, and surround myself with my other children. I would leave for work almost every day in tears, but I had a contract with the producers of *The King and I* and a responsibility to the cast and the audience. However, every night as I sang "Getting to Know You" to the group of darling kids playing the king's children, I missed being with my own.

I wanted my children around me as much as possible, so I brought them to the theater with me when I could, usually just for the matinees. My dressing room was covered with their drawings, art projects, and sometimes their pranks. One night while I was on stage, they soaked about fifteen of my herbal tea bags and tossed them at the ceiling until they stuck. The ceiling was a mosaic of chamomile. It makes you pause and question why we spend so much money on the latest gadget or toy to entertain our children when a three-dollar box of herbal tea works just as well.

There were other days during those weeks when I was so emotionally exhausted I would just sit in my dressing room and stare at the wall. I have always been one of those women who plow through bad circumstances, but this time I felt the bad was overshadowing any good. I would pray, "I don't know how I can go on stage. Please, help me get through this show." Then I would feel a small but growing sense of relief. I felt it was in God's hands.

There are words of gratitude in my journal on the day the doctors told us that Brandon's foot was healing exceptionally well and he would not need the grafting. They assured me that he would have full mobility and only scarring on his ankle, and that because of his young age, he would most likely never remember the injury.

In my work with children's hospitals around the country, I have seen many injured children. The parents stand by helplessly, knowing the situation is out of their hands. They have to trust that the doctors and nurses will care for their children the same way they would care for them if they could. Long after a child is out of pain and back to his or her happy self, a certain look stays in a parent's eyes. I now recognize that look because I've seen it in my own eyes. It's the profound pain of knowing that you are unable to always protect your children. Even as they go off into the world, descending the steps on wobbly legs, accepting the tumbles and shaking off the spills, you stand by, wishing your arms could catch them every time. My little boy might not remember the injury that left the scar on his ankle, but I will never forget it.

The pain of this time for my whole family was not without its blessings. My children became caretakers to one another. They learned quickly about sacrificing their wants to help another in need and grew in reliance on one another. Yet those blessings felt like small consolation and could not heal the deep wound left on my heart.

4

---◆---

Barefoot and Pregnant, That's Me

I have to tell you, I never, ever thought I would do another television show with Donny, especially not twenty years after our first one. Maybe this is a pattern, and we'll be doing another show twenty more years down the road, at ages fifty-nine and sixty-one. I love him, but we both thought we had traveled the *Donny & Marie* road together once in the seventies and that it was best left to retromemories. Our paths had split wide apart after the original show: I went back to my music career, and Donny did his own recording. Just like the song mentioned: I was a little bit country, and he was a little bit rock 'n' roll. There are crossover artists from both of those genres now, but at that time country and rock 'n' roll were as far apart as Kenny G. and Snoop Dogg are today.

It was Dick Clark who brought Donny and me back together for our second show. There's a reason for Dick Clark's longevity in the entertainment business. The man is great insight into the appetite of the American audience.

His career has had a broad influence on almost every generation from the fifties to now. When he visited the *Donny & Marie* soundstage, people in the studio audience ages fifteen to sixty would clamor for his autograph. Dick also has that enviable quality of being able to laugh at himself. For example, one day on *Donny & Marie,* we took the viewing audience on a backstage tour, showing the star-autographed walls, the props, the standby area, photos of guests, and one particular area of interest. I pulled open a door and said, "This is where we keep Dick Clark." There was Dick, standing in a walk-in freezer, apparently stored for preservation purposes. He gave his trademark "thumbs-up" to the camera as smoke from dry ice swirled around him. You've got to love him for his willingness to have fun. (Truthfully, he seemed so at home in there, it made me wonder if that's really how he maintains his youthful look.) I have great respect for Dick's judgment when it comes to television, so when he flew in with John Ferriter, my agent from William Morris, to talk to me at a recording studio where I was working on an album, I listened. I didn't have talk show experience, but I've never had trouble talking! I liked the idea of moving back to L.A. and having a regular daytime job so I could be at home with my kids in the evenings. Doing a television show had its appeal as well. The bottom line is, Dick Clark is a very convincing person.

◆

I remember the first two months of taping *Donny & Marie* ?
one big blur. Going from a rehearsed and scripted Br
way show to a talk show in which the guest or the s
changed every six to ten minutes was a new challe
taped six one-hour shows almost every week.
show would be for the weeks we didn't tape, s
the holidays. Every show had six segments,

different guest or subject matter. That's thirty-six new guests or topics that I had to be knowledgeable enough to talk about every week. It's a fascinating job, but you can never coast.

This was the preparation for one show: I needed to watch film clips from both Jimmy Smits's and Nestor Carbonell's new movies so I knew the subject matter, whether it was comedy or history (often the same thing). I read biographical material on both actors to know what they had done in their career and information on their personal lives. Then I needed to familiarize myself with the demonstration segments: one featured talking with an *InStyle* magazine trend spotter about new colognes preferred by celebrities. The other demo was a just-released computer game, which I had to quickly learn how to play (not as easy as it may sound for a woman who only last year figured out how to program the speed dial on her phone). Diana Krall, the Grammy-winning jazz artist, was also on the same show. I needed to read her bio and listen to her new CD.

For every show, Donny and I did an opening chat, which was a ten-to-twelve-minute segment on a variety of topics: our own lives, events in the news, or human-interest stories. Usually one chat a week consisted of a practical joke that one of us would play on the other. Donny always managed to get me good on one of my more sensitive issues. Once, he and the producer compiled short clips from past shows of me laughing hysterically. Ten clips of me cackling are enough to qualify as torture. I've even received letters from viewers about my laugh, describing it as everything from "obnoxiously nasal" to "a hyena in pain." For their thoughtful comments, I think I'll send those viewers my Laugh-A-Minute Greatest Hits tape!

I loved the fast pace of the job and the unexpected occurrences that kept me on my toes every hour of every tape day. I was chased off stage by giant cockroaches (I'm talking as big as my hand). Tom Green, the MTV madman, cut out the back of my jacket with scissors as the camera rolled (a jacket I had to wear for the next show). I was flipped over the shoulder of a swing dancer and ate a roasted-cricket omelette. Comedian Kathy Griffin said she was sick and tired of women coming on the show and talking about how they had crushes on Donny when they were growing up. She decided to pay attention to me, and laid a big ol' smooch right on my mouth. And I was working with Donny again, but then I was used to working around children in *The King and I,* so that was the easy part of the job. Love ya, Donny!

With all of this going on, by the third month of the show I didn't give much thought to the fact that I was exhausted, until I started waking up in the morning with severe nausea. I bought a home pregnancy test kit. I'm not great at math, but I do know what a plus sign means. It was hard to believe it could be true. I thought my chances of getting pregnant at age thirty-nine were slim to nonexistent. It was clear I had just squeaked into the slim-chance category. The chance was the *only* slim part of this pregnancy.

A couple of weeks later, I gathered all the children together and told them that I was expecting. I told them about writing in my journal years ago that I sensed that sometime in the future I would give birth to a baby boy.

All of the kids were thrilled, but I caught a glimpse of apprehension on the face of my oldest son, Stephen. I'm sure being the firstborn in a family of six children has its drawbacks, including the extra responsibilities of helping to take care of the younger ones. I know he must often think of it as a full-time job, and now I was announcing more unpaid overtime for him.

I was surprised when Stephen decided to go with me and the rest of the kids to UCLA Medical Center for my sonogram appointment in my fourth month. He seemed intensely interested in this procedure. As the nurse ran the wand over my stomach, we watched the image of the baby on the monitor.

"There's the baby's head," I pointed out. "Look at the little arms! What a miracle."

"Great," Stephen said without missing a beat, "but can we get to the important part? This had better be a boy."

He wouldn't admit it right there, but later he revealed that he was scared that this baby would be a girl. "I was worried, Mom," he told me. "I knew if you sensed a boy and wrote about him in your journal and this one happened to be a girl, then there would be at least one more kid in the future."

The next month I announced on the show that I was expecting. I found it hilarious that the tabloids made claims that I had purposely gotten pregnant to increase the ratings of *Donny & Marie*. It would have been more believable to write that I personally visited every Nielsen rating family and rigged their viewing boxes.

As my pregnancy became more visible, I received many e-mails and letters from viewers (especially mothers with young children) saying, "You look so great every day on the show. How do you do it?" It was comforting to hear that they thought I looked great, but I really had very little to do with my appearance. It was all done for me by professional hair, makeup, and wardrobe people. I couldn't have done it on my own, especially considering I was one of those lucky pregnant women who had "morning sickness" morning, noon, and night almost into my fifth month. The only time I had an appetite was late at night, and then I was ravenous. I was like a wolf, hunting by the light of the moon. Only I was hunting by the light of the refrigerator at three in the morning, chomping on the turkey breast and ripping through bags of barbecue potato chips. The family would get up in the morning to see the results of my attack on the deli drawer and my greasy fingerprints on the counter.

By the time I got out of bed in the morning, I couldn't even think about food. A restaurant commercial on TV was enough to send me reeling. I would come into the studio and walk directly into my bathroom. The slightest scent of cologne or eggs or garlic or Donny or whatever I was sensitive to that week was enough to drop me to my knees on the tiles again. Almost every pregnant woman takes her turn "tossing her cookies" in her first few months, but this five-month trek was like having a twenty-four-hour bug for three thousand six hundred hours. I knew for sure how awful I looked when one of the crew members commented on how well my blouse went with my eyes. The blouse was red!

By my fifth month of pregnancy I had so much puffiness in my face that the makeup artist, with paintbrush in hand, would ask me, "Where would you like your cheekbones today?"

The clothes I wore on the show were selected and fitted for me by wardrobe people, Ret Turner and Dina Cerchione. Dina deserves an Emmy for making me presentable on a daily basis through my pregnancy. My body was changing so fast that there was no guarantee that what fit perfectly on Monday could even be zipped up on Thursday.

It was often necessary to pretape a guest on *Donny & Marie*. For example, LeAnn Rimes was out on tour and only able to come to the studio on Tuesday, but she was scheduled for the Thursday show. We did a pretape with her before doing the Tuesday show and saved it to run in the Thursday show. When the Thursday show was actually taped, I would have to be dressed in the same outfit I had worn for the interview with LeAnn on Tuesday. Sometimes during my pregnancy, just the passage of two or three days would mean "alteration city" on my outfit. Laura, my talented seamstress, put in so much overtime keeping up with me that I think she doubled her paycheck as I doubled in size. Sometimes she would have to make quick fixes with a pair of scissors by cutting straight up the back of my blouse then stitching in extra fabric to make it fit. If you catch any reruns of the show, notice that I never turn around during my whole pregnancy. That's because the back of every outfit looks like the description of the coat Dolly Parton's mama made in her song "Coat of Many Colors."

I wore a fuchsia-colored silk blouse under a jacket in a series of different pretapes. It was resurrected so many times that there was no original material left on the back. I don't know how much extra cloth they stitched into the back of that blouse, but at one point in my eighth month, I think someone was cutting up a queen-size sheet to make it work. So you can see just how glamorous showbiz truly is.

On the last day of taping for season one, we were going to have a big fuchsia blouse–burning ceremony. The executive producer, Charlie Cook, said, "I never want to see you wear that blouse again." He was reserving first place in line to light a match to the thing. When the time came, though, I found I couldn't burn it. The blouse had become a timeline of the pregnancy and almost a quilt of the *Donny & Marie* show. We would look at the back of the blouse and say: "Look, here's the two inches we added for the Tony Curtis show, and here's an extension of material from when Whoopi Goldberg came on. Here's the duct tape we used when Fergie made an appearance." My daughters begged me to save the silver lamé insert that was sewn in for our show with 'N Sync.

I probably should have burned the blouse and done something dramatic with it, like scatter the ashes on Cindy

Crawford's front porch in an act of alteration protest. Did she *have* to be pregnant at the exact same time I was? In fact, she had her baby the same day I did, and they weighed the same. Unfortunately, that's all we had in common. She went through her entire pregnancy with only a cute little tummy, looking like she'd tucked a bulky sweater into a pair of jeans. I thought about having a restraining order taken out against her so if we ended up at any of the same events, she'd have to stay at least five hundred yards away from me. That way we could never be photographed side by side. I could see the caption on that photo of Cindy and me now: "The gorgeous and the gorged."

One of my favorite things about doing the television show was having a great staff, like Ret, Dina, and Laura, who would go to any length to make something work. Almost every person I worked with on the show had great enthusiasm and an even greater ability to adapt to whatever needed to happen to get the show on the air. Adaptability is one of the most treasured traits in television because during every show at least one thing is going to fall apart or change from the original production plan. Whether it was patching together a blouse, setting up an Easter egg hunt, or turning a cooking demonstration set into a rock 'n' roll stage in a matter of minutes, the *Donny & Marie* staff always made it look easy. And not only easy but fun! They would go to any extremes for a good laugh. During my seventh and eighth months of pregnancy, my stomach was so large I would have to sit out some of the more physical demonstrations, like exercise and dance segments. Even standing felt like physical exertion by the last month. The writers, Marcia and Ed, and the prop guys, Mike and Robert, designed books for me to read, sitting on the couch, while Donny sweated away on the next new aerobic workout. The books were oversized, with huge titles on their covers like *The Baby Ate My Brain* and

Chocolate Soup for the Third-Trimester Soul. One of my favorites was *Control Your Bladder, Control Your Life.* The last one had a lot of truth to it. When a comedian came on, I knew I would only be safe if I sprinted to the bathroom right before the segment. During my eighth month and in three-inch heels, I'm sure this looked ridiculous.

I found the pace of the talk show to be similar to my show at home with my kids. Adaptability is also one of the most important attributes in parenting. Every day with your baby is like producing a show, except there isn't a whole crew available to help you get it together when everything comes apart at the last minute. Mothers do the jobs of many. Our job description in a paycheck world would be reason to hire a whole crew of people. In one of the opening chats on *Donny & Marie,* we talked about a poll taken by a research group that broke down the job duties of a mother. The list included cook, chauffeur, nurse, tutor, dog walker, counselor, housekeeper, and repair person, among others. If you add up the average income for these positions, a stay-at-home mother's salary should be $500,000 a year.

The media try to make the job of mother appear to be a breeze, a mindless luxury job. We are bombarded by commercials starring moms with huge smiles and plates full of fresh-baked after-school treats for the whole soccer team. There are images of women in beautifully lit rooms with silky curtains blowing in the breeze, rocking infants in polished cherry-wood chairs. One of my favorites is the ad featuring the woman with long, flowing hair falling around her shoulders, wearing full makeup and a cashmere sweater while bathing her baby. Oh, come on. I can only imagine what she dresses like when she hauls the garbage cans to the curb.

Seven months into my pregnancy, I was asked by Dick Clark to be a presenter at the Academy of Country Music

Awards. Finding evening wear in maternity styles is not the easiest thing to do, but my great wardrobe people brought in a lovely black knee-length dress with beading around the hem and neckline. I changed into it right after we finished taping for the day while a limo waited to take me to the awards.

My two toddlers, Brandon and Brianna, had been with me that day at work, playing in the little nursery off my dressing room. Suddenly, Brandon, who was then two and a half, ran into the dressing room crying hysterically. When I bent down to take him in my arms, he buried his face in my neck and proceeded to leave a runny-nose trail across my entire shoulder and down my sleeve. We all looked at one another in horror, and Dina, the wardrobe person, momentarily looked like she would cry. Then we started talking about what it would be like for me to show up at the awards ceremony with (excuse the image) baby boogers across my shoulder, and laughed. In L.A., most people get held up by traffic. I run late because of a runny nose. And when I arrive, you won't have to look long to find a mini handprint someplace on what I'm wearing.

That's reality for most of us. Or at least the moms I know. You should see me after I've been with the kids all weekend. I'm grateful if I can look in a mirror long enough to comb my hair and make sure my shoes match . . . or that I'm wearing shoes at all.

On one typically hectic morning, after getting the kids off to school with the right homework in their backpacks and the babies changed and fed, I jumped into the car, threw my briefcase on the seat next to me, and drove away in a hurry. I tried to use the forty-five-minute drive in to the studio to mentally prepare for the shows that day. About halfway into the trip, I realized I didn't have any shoes on. I didn't even have any with me in the car to put on. It was too late to turn back, so I drove in barefoot. I was hoping I could just sneak into the studio and find a pair in my dressing room. Of course, that had to be a day when a coffee cart was parked right outside the stage door, and I was forced to walk by several staff members waiting in line. I just smiled and waved when one of them called out to me, "Too bad Mormons don't drink coffee. It usually makes you alert enough to remember to put shoes on."

Later that morning, I thought perhaps I had been subconsciously hoping I would be pulled over by the police, because it's against the law to drive barefoot in California. Then maybe I could have been thrown in jail for twenty-four hours and caught up on some sleep.

♦

As amazing as the tricks are for looking good on television, the advertising and publishing worlds can be another dimension altogether. How can women feel anything but substandard when compared to the perfection the media parades before us? Our self-esteem can be punished every time we flip through a fashion magazine, because the message on the page is: You should be able to have a baby and beautiful skin and a flat tummy and thick eyelashes and a career and drive a sports car and meet your man in a four-star restaurant and wear four-inch heels with polished toenails . . . and . . . and . . . and. What mothers are they modeling these ads after? These days, human perfection can be manufactured, especially in photographs. What you see is not always what's really there. I've learned that perfect skin can come from three coats of makeup and some magic with an airbrush. And once in a while, the touch-up is on more than the face.

Donny and I had to shoot our publicity photos for season two at the very end of season one. In the photo the publicity department chose for our billboards, I'm sitting on an ottoman with my head leaning on my hand. Donny is seated on the floor at my feet. (I'll let that one go by.) I look very postbaby sleek, dressed in black. Okay, now for the reality of that photograph. I was really in my last month of pregnancy. I'm leaning forward with my head in my hand because my belly was so big I could barely sit up straight. Technology is mind-boggling. My pregnant stomach was digitally removed from the photograph, some extra weight was taken off my back, and they even took some puffiness from my face. (I would try this at home, but I don't fit in the scanner.)

Personally, I gave up trying to keep it all together after my second child. I invested in some longer jackets to cover it all up and have never looked back. It's too much extra effort to maintain a perfect image, and I'd rather spend the time having fun with my children. My kids will always come before cosmetics or cars or my career because the picture I have of my family in my head has nothing to do with looking put together and everything to do with actually being together.

My baby is the only adoring audience that really counts. And he's not critical at all of how I look, what I drive, or even if the dishes are done. He could care less if I've managed to put on mascara. He just wants to sit on my lap and have me read *One Fish Two Fish Red Fish Blue Fish* . . . again and again and again.

5

◆

Fine. Great.

Three days after we wrapped the first season of *Donny & Marie* and eight months into my pregnancy, I caught a plane to Orlando to participate in the seventeenth annual Children's Miracle Network (CMN) broadcast. The June broadcast raises millions of dollars for the Children's Miracle Network, a charity that actor John Schneider and I cofounded almost two decades ago. What began as a good idea has grown into a phenomenal organization that helps hospitals to help more than 14 million kids every year. Doctors, nurses, social workers, medical technicians, and volunteers work to create miracles every day by giving children a chance at a quality life. CMN allows children's hospitals located throughout North America to have an open-door policy, serving any child who needs medical attention, regardless of the family's ability to pay.

The stories we feature on the CMN broadcast about the Miracle Kids, children who have received help, are inspiring. It's tough for anyone to remain unmoved after witnessing their inexhaustible spirit and the incredible effort of thousands of people who volunteer their time to help these children triumph over disease, birth defects, and injury.

The time I spend working with Children's Miracle Network and visiting the children every year is an absolute pleasure and joy. I've never missed an annual broadcast, and though my family and friends were telling me that I was burning the candle at both ends by going to this one, my heart would not stay quiet and allow me to stay home. Here I was, carrying a healthy baby and with six other children who were also thriving and in good health. How could I set aside the hardships of parents with children who struggle with daily existence simply because I was tired and in my third trimester of pregnancy? My doctor in Los Angeles gave me the okay to go and cleared me to fly because I checked out fine.

Everything went smoothly until mid-morning on the second day of the broadcast, when I started to feel vague contractions. They weren't close together, but I could definitely tell they were contractions. I consulted with an OB-GYN connected with CMN who was at the broadcast. He listened as I described what I was experiencing and then suggested that I get off my feet and rest in bed for a couple of hours. If it was actual labor, the contractions would continue to increase, but only time would tell.

Every year, to wrap up the event, I sit on stage surrounded by the Miracle Kids and sing "Thank God for Kids," which was a hit for the Oak Ridge Boys. We usually schedule this right before the final tally on the tote board. I didn't want to leave without doing the song, so I told a couple of the producers about my situation. They made a quick schedule change, and I performed the song three hours earlier than usual, hugged the kids and the volunteers good-bye, and then, with regret, headed off to the hotel to rest.

As soon as I lay down the contractions eased up and then stopped. I felt that everything would be fine and I wanted to be with my kids and near my own doctor, so I started getting ready to fly home. Brian called ahead to make alternate flight reservations, but he also wanted me to check in again with the OB-GYN at the broadcast. The doctor thought I had experienced a short bout of false labor, since the contractions had stopped hours before. He said it was safe for me to fly but suggested that once I was home, I stop to see my own doctor at UCLA Medical Center.

Following the flight, we made an appointment to meet up with my L.A. doctor in his office. He did some tests, including drawing some amniotic fluid to see if the baby was fully developed. The doctor confirmed that the baby was not ready to be born and that the contractions had been false labor. He estimated that the baby was at least a couple of weeks away from delivery and advised me to go home and rest.

I was thinking, "Rest? That's going to be a challenge."

You know how you can feel really, really full after eating Thanksgiving dinner? It hurts to sit up, you're too full to go for a walk, and lying down makes you feel like a beanbag chair with someone curled up on top of you. That's what I was feeling like twenty-four hours a day.

If I had known it would be another four weeks before this baby arrived, I think I would have just tumbled into a hammock in the backyard and started shouting out orders. "I'll get up when the baby gets out. In the meantime, run a root beer float IV out here to the hammock. And I like my popcorn buttered, with salt." Talk about your cravings—I wanted to salt my toothpaste.

Once we knew that the baby wasn't ready to be born, Brian decided it was a good time to finish producing an album he was working on in Utah. I understood he was on a deadline and I felt okay with the decision. I knew he was less than a two-hour flight away and could come home quickly if something happened. I was also relaxed about it because I wasn't handling everything on my own. We had two young nannies, Jill and Melissa, who came to the house every day to assist me with the children's schedules and in keeping track of the little ones. I think toddlers can sense when Mommy can't catch up to them anymore, and mine were smart enough to take full advantage of that. I had to bring in a relief team.

Even with help during the day, it was hard for me to physically rest because I couldn't mentally rest at all. Knowing that *Donny & Marie* was coming back for a second season, we thought it would be more practical to buy a house in L.A. than to continue renting. We had found a perfect-sized home with enough bedrooms (not as easy as you might think with seven kids), on a cul-de-sac, which I loved, with lots of neighborhood kids. I wouldn't have to worry about street traffic every time the kids went out the front door, just the constant traffic jam of teenagers and tots coming through the front door, steering for the kitchen, and cleaning out a week's worth of groceries in one trip.

I'm sure I don't have to tell anyone the headaches that come with trying to pack and move a household, but when you can't really bend over, lift, carry, or even get a good, deep breath because of the size of your stomach, then it's a real challenge. To pack something, I had to drop it into a box from waist high, which was pretty rough on my china.

◆

I may have slowed down, but the baby hadn't. He was really active because I was carrying extra fluid due to the condition of my kidneys. The baby could literally swim in my belly when he was full term. (Maybe I should have swallowed a penny that he could dive for.) To keep him occupied, and me as well, I made up a little game to play with him. I would tap one part of my tummy, and in a matter of seconds he would bump up against that spot. Then I would pick another place to tap, and he would move over to bump into that area. My little ones loved playing this game with the baby too. If the older kids were playing their music too loud, he would tap against my stomach as if to say, "Hey, keep it down out there." And of course, with his Osmond genes, the tapping was right on the beat.

The water weight gain put extra strain and pressure on my hips and lower back, and it got increasingly difficult to be comfortable at all. The only real relief was to soak in a warm bath; that way the baby and I could both swim. I would light some candles and then float in the bubbles, holding my hands over my tummy and talking to my baby. I would tell him how much I looked forward to his arrival and how much his sisters and brothers loved him. I also requested that since my other labors had always been more than twenty hours long, when he decided to make his grand entrance, "Please, make it fast!"

At my next weekly checkup, the doctor could see how uncomfortable I was. I was also showing symptoms of toxemia, which caused concern. Following some tests, he suggested that labor could be induced, since the baby was now fully developed. I called Brian, who said he would catch the first possible flight in from Utah and bring his mother, Georgia.

I was thrilled with this prospect of delivering because I was having a hard time even climbing the stairs to the second floor of our house. We decided to proceed, so the nurse administered Pitocin through an IV, which began the contractions. My girlfriends Patty and Shawn, not wanting me to be alone at the hospital, arrived soon after with the atmosphere: candles and essential oils for aromatherapy, and soothing music for the background. My personal manager, Karl, came from his office in L.A. to lend support. I called home to let the kids know their baby brother was on his way and one of the nannies arrived a short time later with the bag I had packed for the hospital. We were all thinking that the baby's birthday was just hours away. It ended up being like a surprise birthday party where the guest of honor never shows up, because twenty hours (that's the big two-oh!) of labor went by and still no baby. The reason I remember it was twenty whole hours is that I went through every minute without an epidural. None. Zippo. Did you hear me say "Ow"?

Unpredictably, in the twentieth hour the contractions were coming farther apart instead of intensifying. The doctor ordered the Pitocin IV to be stopped and told me, "This baby doesn't seem to want to make an appearance today. He must have a different date in mind. We'll keep an eye on the toxemia symptoms, but you should go home and take it easy."

I felt terrible, as if I had let everyone down. They had put their schedules on hold, and I hadn't delivered, literally. I couldn't believe that I was going to check out of the hospital without a baby in my arms after all of that, but the doctor told us that this had happened before with other women and it was nothing to be concerned about. He did think we should do a sonogram to make sure the baby was fine.

I remember thinking, "I'm going to have my work cut out for me with this kid. Even in the womb, he has a mind of his own." I didn't realize how right I was until a short time later, when the baby sent me a message over the sonogram screen. The image showed him resting serenely in his quiet personal spa with one of his little hands stretched toward the viewer. We all started laughing because his middle finger stood alone, as if to say, "I didn't really appreciate that last twenty hours and I'll come out when I'm good and ready."

I just sat there grinning and thought, "Oh, brother. This kid isn't going to leave home until he's forty-five."

Brian was in the final stages of finishing his album project. (At least one of us was in the final stages of producing something!) So he flew back to Utah the next morning and his mom stayed with me to help out.

This is my first strong memory of starting to feel upset and anxious about the course of the pregnancy, and I would say now that it may have been the precursor of my depression. I couldn't help but feel pressure about giving birth. The longer I stayed pregnant, the less time I had to get in shape to go back to work, and remembering how it was with my other pregnancies, I knew it would take concentrated effort to exercise and get the weight off. It wouldn't be easy at age forty to lose the sixty pounds I had gained. I was concerned with the move to the new house, and I had job commitments starting in a month, including personal appearances that had been planned over a year ago and would be hard to reschedule once I started back at the show for season two. The phone started ringing nonstop with people wanting to know if the baby had arrived and when I would be ready to go back to work.

My hips and lower back had so much weight-gain pressure that I couldn't move without wincing in pain. I was barely sleeping two consecutive hours because no matter what position I tried, the pressure cut off my circulation, making my legs and feet go numb. As soon as I found a comfortable position for my hips, the heartburn would kick in. Almost nightly, I would go out to the kids' swing set in the backyard and sit in a saddle swing. The way I was squeezed by it took the pressure off my hips and relieved some of the pain.

One morning after breakfast, I was standing at the kitchen sink chatting with my mother-in-law, Georgia.

I could tell she felt bad for me. She tried to keep me upbeat and cheerful by saying, "This kid's stubborn, just like his dad. It's going to take a miracle to get him out. What we need is a sign, so we don't feel stressed about when he's going to be ready to be born."

As soon as she finished voicing that thought, a bird flew full speed into the kitchen window right behind her head. It startled both of us, but I'm sure not as much as it did the little bird, which lay stunned momentarily, then flapped its wings and flew off.

Georgia jumped up from the kitchen table and said while laughing, "That's it. That's our sign!"

The thought of a bird's smacking into the window being a sign made me start laughing hysterically too. What was the message? "The baby isn't coming because the stork's been knocked unconscious?" The more I thought about it the harder I laughed, until I was crouched over, shrieking.

My mother-in-law then pointed to the floor and said, "Look, Marie. Your water broke!"

Could it be true? Was today the day? Was it really my sign? Nope. No way. No such luck. With my stomach as big as it was, I couldn't feel anything below my ribs. I was laughing so hard my bladder had packed up and gone on vacation because it couldn't take the job pressure anymore. Embarrassing, yes, but the laughter got me through the day.

This is a prime example of my core belief that humor helps us survive. Even in our most painful, vulnerable, unattractive, or embarrassing moments, the ability to laugh can be the lifeline that pulls us through.

When the Fourth of July weekend came around, I gave up worrying and decided the baby was not paying any attention to my schedule whatsoever. I was just going to have to relax and let it happen when it would. Brian thought I should get out of the house because I couldn't leave the packing for the move alone and the disorder was making me uneasy. He suggested we go to our house in Utah. That way the kids could be with their relatives and I could be near Brian while he worked over the holiday. The nannies said they would drive the car up if I wanted to fly with the kids.

Again, I called my doctor, who thought it would be fine to fly. Maybe it wasn't the wisest choice I've ever made, but I did want to be near my parents and Brian, and the kids were so excited. Georgia was tired of mopping and wanted to go home. She called her airline and took a flight out that night. The next morning the rest of us went to the airport and bought the last seven seats available. Somehow, they arranged for us all to be seated together in the back of the plane. I'll never forget the faces of the other passengers as we made our way down the aisle. Me, ready to burst, trailed by a sixteen-year-old boy carrying two full diaper bags, then five children under age twelve. Some people actually went pale, though I'm not sure if it was from the size of my brood or the size of my tummy. They probably thought they were in for an eventful plane ride.

My children have traveled all over the world with me, and it's important to me that they try not to impose on anyone with their actions. When I was a kid touring with my family, my mother had us each pack what she called a "busy box." It was an activity kit with puzzles, games, books, crafts, and small toys or whatever else would entertain us. I've carried on the tradition with my own children, and though they can have their moments, my kids are patient when it comes to traveling and usually conscientious about their airplane manners. When we landed in Salt Lake City, the other passengers decided to let the pregnant woman and her posse get off first. As we walked down the aisle, someone started clapping for the kids' good behavior, and then suddenly all the passengers joined the round of applause. Brianna, my youngest, did the Queen Mother wave down the aisle. The applause was a sweet gesture, but now the younger ones expect it every time they fly.

We have had our house in Provo, Utah, throughout all the touring, Broadway runs, and our time in L.A. for *Donny & Marie*. It's impossible to predict how long any tour or television show will last, so it's nice to always have a place to call home. We bought the house when we only had three children, and it's perfect for a family of five. It's a little more challenging for a family of nine. There isn't a bedroom, except Brain's and mine, without wall-to-wall beds.

Even so, everyone seemed to be thrilled to be home in Utah. The nannies arrived in the car a day later, and the Fourth of July atmosphere was in full swing. The kids and their cousins took off to go swimming, hiking, biking, and boating on the lake. I wished I could participate, but just moving from the couch to the kitchen was wearing me out.

On our third day in Utah, I began to feel great pain around my abdominal area. This time it didn't feel like contractions, so I was anxious. Brian was taking a day off and had left the house early to take the kids water-skiing about forty-five minutes away. Worried, I placed a call to the doctor who had delivered my other babies in Utah and explained to him the history of this pregnancy. He requested I meet him immediately at the hospital for a sonogram. When he looked at the screen his face took on a look of concern, which didn't make me feel relieved. He explained that the reason for my pain was that the baby had moved into breech position, which could mean birth complications. Unless the baby turned back into a head-down position, a C-section delivery was my only option. He told me I should go home to rest and call him the next day.

The next morning, the kids were anxious to go out on the boat again. I didn't want to hold up the plans for the weekend, so I told Brian to go ahead with the kids since nothing seemed to be changing for me, and it was pointless for them all to sit at home. With a cell phone in his pocket, Brian loaded the kids in the car and took off for the lake. Around noon I began to feel the same abdominal pain I had felt the day before. When it continued to increase in intensity over the next thirty minutes I placed a call to my Utah doctor.

My doctor suggested that the baby was possibly turning again into the head-down position in the womb, but he felt I should meet him at the hospital to be examined to see if a C-section was necessary.

Despite my feelings of distress at the prospect of having a C-section, when the doctor told me he would make the arrangements to have me checked into the hospital right away, I said, "Fine. Great." I wanted to cry out, "I'm frightened. Everyone has left me. I can't do this alone," but instead I said, "Fine. Great." I didn't let on that I was scared. After all, I had given birth before, and I was too proud to admit to any fear.

You would think that by the time the doctor had informed me of the possible complications with the birth, I would have raised the white flag of surrender and asked someone to help me instead of pretending I was fine. But the self-reliant side of me still insisted that I could handle this news and that I could work it all out. I called Brian to tell him I was being admitted. I could hear my family having great fun in the background. I felt terrible, as if I were ruining their day. I told Brian to come to the hospital when he could. I tried not to sound urgent, but I really needed him to be there. I knew that by the time he got the boat docked, the kids dried off and changed, and drove home, it would be almost two hours later.

After I checked in, I remember sitting on the edge of the hospital bed, knowing that my baby would be born in Utah, perhaps before the day ended. I was alone, but even worse, I had never felt more lonely. There were no candles, no soft music, no faces of friends and family surrounding my bed. My parents were a three-hour car trip away, and my husband, his family, and our kids were all out in the sunshine on the lake. I was at the hospital, drowning in the image that I had worked so hard for everyone to buy hook, line, and sinker: Marie is always "fine."

6

It's Independence Day for
America, Labor Day for Me

Matthew R. Blosil was placed in my arms at two o'clock
in the morning on July 6. He was a remarkable miracle, one
small cell, divided millions of times to grow into another life
that would take its place in human history. A newborn child
is all possibilities . . . the future in a seven-pound, eleven-
ounce package. I was elated. I felt overwhelming joy from
the top of my head to . . . just above my waist. I was still
receiving medication through an epidural in my spine. I
couldn't feel anything below my middle. Now that's my idea
of natural childbirth. I think it's perfectly natural to not
want to feel anything after countless contractions.

The doctor had determined that the baby had flipped
again and was in position, so a C-section wasn't necessary. I
breathed a sigh of relief because I didn't have the time to
rest and recover properly from having an incision.

Brian and my two older daughters, Jessica and Rachael,
were there. I also had invited Brian's only sister, Kathy, and
both of our mothers to be present in the birthing room. The

doctor, the nurses, and the anesthesiologist made it a room-ful. It was like being at a party where everyone crowds into the kitchen and you want to shout, "Can I just get a glass of water?"

My girls, then twelve and ten, had asked to be there when Matthew was born. At first they stood near my shoulders, excited and ready to greet their new little brother. Then, as one hour became two, then three, then six, they curled up in chairs along the side of the room. I wanted them to witness the miracle of birth, but after a while the expression on their faces said, "When is this going to be over?" I thought it would be a good life lesson for them to understand that the best things come through hard work and sometimes pain. I think they dozed off through much of the "hard work" part, though. I was wishing I could join them.

My father and Brian's father waited together in the entryway behind a privacy curtain. My mother told me later that my father broke down in tears right after Matthew was born. During the births of all nine of his kids, my father, like all men of that time, had been banished to the waiting room. He told my mother that he was moved because even with so many children and grandchildren, he had never heard the very first cry of a newborn.

My mother, on the other hand, was quite familiar with the first cry, not only from her own nine, but from a number of her grandchildren. Matthew was number fifty-two, so she now had one grandchild for each week of the year. I considered buying her one of those charm necklaces with the little boy and girl figures for each grandchild but had to let go of that idea. She'd never be able to stand up straight with fifty-two birthstones hanging around her neck.

My fatigue from the delivery started to crash over me soon afterward. I wanted to rest. Everyone stayed only long enough to welcome the baby, and then the nurse took him to be cleaned up while I was rolled away to a regular room. I think I fell sound asleep before I was even moved off the gurney. They must have just tossed me from the gurney onto the bed, because I have no memory of getting in on my own. They probably could have propped me up in the cleaning supplies closet and I would have slept just as soundly. By that time my hair was looking like the working end of a mop anyway, so I would have blended right in.

When I woke again early that morning I expected to feel achy and sore. To my great surprise, I was feeling terrific. I got up and took a shower and washed my hair. I remember thinking, "This is great. I must have really stayed in shape while doing the first season of the talk show, because I feel better than I did when I gave birth years ago."

The baby was in a bassinet in the room with me for the sake of privacy. It had already been leaked that I had been admitted to the hospital in labor, and it was only a matter of time before the photographers started to show up.

Having those first few minutes alone with my baby that morning was wonderful. I wanted to memorize everything about him on this first day of his life. My heart was captured by his tiny fingers wrapped around my thumb and his upper lip, which arched in the middle the same way Stephen's did when he was born. I whispered in his perfect little ear how happy I was that he was here with me. I tried to preserve the moment as long as I could and give him a gentle introduction to the world. And then, it seemed as though the whole world came by to introduce itself to him.

Within the first hour of my waking up, many large flower arrangements arrived bearing congratulatory notes from family and friends. Then my own family came to see the baby. My two toddlers crawled into bed with me to check out the new family member, and soon the string of other visitors started up and continued nonstop for hours. I was thrilled to have my loved ones around me, some of whom I hadn't seen in the full year that we had lived in L.A. They were all people I loved, and each was excited to see the baby and share in my joy.

About mid-morning I could feel my system starting to rebel. My stomach area became painful, and my lack of rest was catching up with me quickly. My "early bird" enthusiasm from five hours before was now more like "the worm who had been caught." I felt like I had been stretched to my limit.

I was starting to tire of the noise and confusion as more and more visitors, flowers, balloons, and candy filled the room. It's not that anyone overstayed his or her welcome, or that I didn't appreciate their support, it's just that I had no chance to rest or even take a break. Besides all the people in the room, I was taking phone call after phone call from my friends and business associates from around the country.

Foremost in my mind was my concern at how many people were holding the baby. I was worried that he was being exposed to too many germs before his brand-new little immune system could kick in. I estimated that he was held by at least fifty people in a span of four hours. How's that for a birthday party?

My Utah neighbor and good friend LuAnn Samuelian came to visit, and after seeing how many people were in the room and spilling out into the hallway, she made her way to my bedside for a quick hello. As she leaned down to hug me she said, "You should be sleeping right now. Do you want me to ask people to leave so you can rest?"

I wanted to accept her offer, but how could I? Looking at the faces of my friends and family and how delighted they were to see the baby, I didn't have the heart to ask for time alone. I could only smile and shake my head, even though I was ready to burst into tears.

That evening, I felt sad thinking how unsettling the day must have been for my baby. My kids are used to having a lot of people around, but I didn't feel it was the first thing Matthew needed to experience. Brian could see that I was overtired and, concerned that my room number had been too available to anyone who asked, arranged to have me moved to a room with more privacy. We decided to limit visitors the next day by inventing a code name visitors would have to use at the front desk to be given my room number. I felt bad about it because visiting was such a sweet show of support from my friends, but the pace of the day's "open house" had been too much for me to handle.

◆

When visiting hours were long over, they pushed me in a wheelchair down the hallway into a new room. I'm sure it must have looked like a going-out-of-business sale for a florist shop, as hospital aides and nurses carried about twenty-five bouquets down the hallway. Or, more likely, it probably looked like a funeral procession, because by that time I looked like death warmed over.

I can't begin to tell you how good it felt to finally be able to rest alone for a couple of hours. I just wanted to cuddle my baby and fall asleep. Outside, the rest of the country was resting up from their Independence Day holiday; inside, I was resting up from Labor Day.

That night, I had a dream that made no sense to me until I looked at it in retrospect. I was in a house that seemed to be mine. It was a place that I would love to live in: a large, white clapboard house with huge windows spilling sunlight onto beautiful hardwood floors. Fresh flowers adorned the tables. It was perfect, but I couldn't stay there. I had to see what was downstairs. I walked down the steps into a dark, windowless room. The air was still and cool. I peered into the dimly lit room, curious about what it held. I could see shelves full of old books and large, rusted metal sculptures hanging from the ceiling. The heads of deer and other hunted game were mounted on the wood-paneled walls. I wasn't afraid; in fact, I wanted to be there. It felt like a haven where I could be creative and adventurous and could hide from the world.

I remembered this dream about six months later and shared it with the counselor who talked with me about postpartum depression. I now believe that it was a glimpse of my true self wanting to escape the Marie Osmond world I had created for myself. I saw the dream as wanting to free the woman who does what she thinks is the right or helpful thing for everyone else first. I felt it was my subconscious telling me that it was time to accept that I couldn't keep up that life anymore. The illusion could no longer cover the reality. There were other parts of me that needed attention, things deep inside that I had never allowed to have a voice.

I don't think I could have predicted, lying in that hospital bed, that I would have to leave the path that my life had been on, the one that would have kept everyone else happy. I didn't know that my future would hold months of wandering, lost to myself, as though through dense woods, struggling to return to safety but only going in deeper. I had no warning that the first day of my baby's life would be my last day on that path. I would never walk it again. I would only emerge when I stopped to clear a new way.

7

Honorable Discharge

I had no choice except to sneak out of the hospital in the middle of the night. No one expects a mother with a new-born to check out at three-thirty in the morning. That is exactly why I had to do it.

The word had spread that I had been admitted to the hospital and given birth to a healthy baby boy. One of my friends who visited told me that the press and curiosity seekers had set up camp at every single exit, anxious and determined to get that first photo of me with my baby. The nursing staff was especially on guard, because even people who were visiting other patients were roaming the halls with cameras, hoping to snap a photo.

I know that people are curious about the private life behind a celebrity image. I appreciate my fans, whom I consider to be friends, and their dedication. I tell them as much about my personal life as I feel comfortable doing. I know the ones who truly care about me have always respected my privacy.

But the tabloids are a different story. Each of the tabloids wanted the first picture, and one of them even offered my business manager, Allen Finlinson, forty thousand dollars for a snapshot. He reported to me that he told them, "Not a dime less than forty-five thousand," and I came back with, "You should have asked for an even fifty." We both laughed.

I said, "Allen, I know you would never consider it. Even if a photo somehow happened to leak to the tabloids and you coincidentally happened to be driving a new BMW next week, I would never, ever suspect you. Besides, you'd need a good car to go *job hunting!*"

Allen has been working with me since I was a teenager. He was the guy who helped me lace my ice skates on the original show, and now he's my business manager. I figure tight laced is tight laced, right? We have hundreds of funny stories of being on the road together, which grow each year from exaggeration. No one can remember what happened originally, since there have been many interesting twists and characters added to every tale. He met and married my wardrobe person, Breta, who also toured with me and now helps me with costume designs for my dolls. Eighteen years later, she still looks exactly the same. Allen, on the other hand, has lost most of his hair. I'm pretty sure I did that to him.

The secret code name we had established seemed to be helping to give me more privacy and limit the number of visitors so I could rest. Unfortunately, it was so secret that some of my brothers didn't even know it. I must have gotten tired of phoning. It's a long list.

Donny and I grew up and performed with five of the hardest-working men in show business—my brothers. Alan, who has retired due to multiple sclerosis, was the group leader. Wayne, Merrill, Jay, and Jimmy continue to perform as the Osmond Brothers to standing-room-only shows at the

Osmond Family Theater in Branson, Missouri, and other venues throughout this country and Europe. Despite our very distinct personalities (some of us are case studies, believe me), we absolutely love and cherish one another. All of us love our spouses and adore children, as proven by the size of each of our families, so a new baby is always cause for us to get together.

My brother Merrill was not too happy when he was unable to see his brand-new nephew. It wasn't like he didn't try. He came to the hospital to see me, dressed up and looking sharp, his beard clipped and his salt-and-pepper hair (mostly salt) all in place. He stopped in the lobby and asked for the room number of his sister. The receptionist, as directed, asked if he knew the code name.

He had no idea what it was, so he tried to convince the receptionist that he was an Osmond, even trying to prove it by smiling to show the trademark mouthful of teeth. She gave him the once-over, stopping on the salt-and-pepper hair, and said, "Look, pal. I'm a big fan of the Osmonds, and you're not one of them." After attempting to reach me on my busy cell phone to get the code name, he gave up trying and left. A short time later Donny showed up, wearing running pants and a T-shirt, his hair disheveled. He looked as if he had just been ejected from a twenty-four-hour fitness center after being there for twenty-five hours. He didn't know the code name either, but the receptionist did recognize him. She gave him the room number, but not before asking him to sing a couple of lines of "Puppy Love."

As tired as I was, I felt the need to look good for the family and friends who would be stopping by to see the baby during my hospital stay. I'm sure I imposed this on myself, but I could tell I looked drained and tired. A new baby is a happy occasion, and as usual I wanted to look that way. My family was also taking pictures, and with us, one bad photo can resurface a dozen times. So I washed my face and put on makeup as soon as I woke up the second morning.

Two women from hospital housekeeping came in to clean up my room at six A.M. I know hospitals run around the clock, but please, at six A.M.? They both looked rather disappointed and were whispering to each other, so I asked, "Is something wrong?"

Finally, one admitted, "We were just hoping to see what Marie Osmond looks like without makeup."

Sounding as offended as I could, I said, "I haven't put any on . . ." (I let them sweat a little) ". . . in the last fifteen minutes." Then I offered, "You're not going to catch me without makeup, but if you want, you two can see what my hair looks like matted down from the pillow."

"It's not the same thing," one explained, ignoring my display of the back of my hair with a shrug. "Everybody in here has bed head."

I loved my doctor, nurses, and the staff at the hospital, actually both hospitals—Utah and Los Angeles. The nurses really took good care of me and also did an excellent job helping to protect my privacy. Theirs is a job few of us can comprehend. Every day they comfort the hurting, helpless, and grieving, as well as supporting new life, both through birth and a return to health. Each hour of the day they deal with people who are in crisis or going through major life changes and who are full of concerns and questions. I'm so impressed with how generous most of them are with affection and their sense of humor. If this doesn't sell you on the virtues of nursing, just remember: When you go in to deliver, they're the ones who give out the painkillers. Got it?

After my doctor had given the "thumbs-up" on my discharge, I had to figure out a way to leave without the tabloid photographers seeing me. It seemed the only way to avoid the photographers was to make a predawn run for it.

The doctors said that I had recovered enough physically and that the baby and I were free of complications. Medically, this may have been true, but I instinctively knew that I was not ready to leave. I wanted to stay in the hospital to rest and have someone take care of me and the baby. I even craved hospital food. That tells you something.

Call it what you will: woman's intuition, almost-age-forty exhaustion, or just the idea of dealing with preteens who wanted to get tattoos and the ever-ready energy of a toddler on a fruit-roll-up high, I did not feel ready to go home. I didn't want to have to sneak out of the hospital. I wanted to sneak back between the blankets and sleep for another nine months, until my body could get back to normal. That seemed like the right amount of recovery time: nine months to produce, nine months to reduce.

Thoughts of returning to my regular life made my head spin as I got dressed and packed my bags (including the two under my eyes) at three in the morning. I felt extremely tired and got dizzy if I moved too quickly. I brushed it off as being up too early and not having had enough sleep.

I'd always brought my new babies home from the hospital in (no, I'm not going to say a suitcase) a little outfit and receiving blanket that I choose just for them. I had saved the tiny little booties, matching outfits, and silky blankets that each of my other children were wrapped up in when they were first brought home, putting them away for them to see when they got older.

One of my best friends, Patty Leoni, had bought a darling receiving outfit that I wanted Matthew to wear home. It was a cream-colored newborn nightie with blue satin trim, a sweet little matching cap, and a satin blanket.

Before going into the hospital, I had washed and ironed the little outfit perfectly and laid it carefully between sheets of tissue paper on top of my clothes in the suitcase. Over the

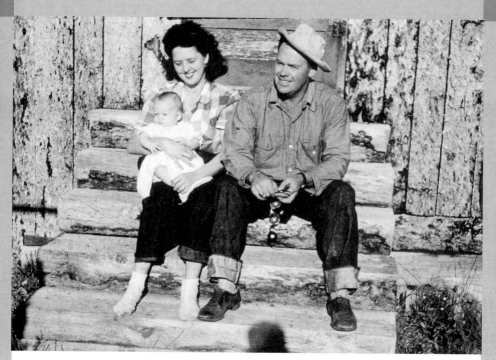

My mother and father with child number eight—and their only girl!
(*Osmond Family Archive*)

Just one of the hundreds of times I waited backstage for my brothers to finish performing. We would all pack up the bus and move on to the next show in the next city.
(*Osmond Family Archive*)

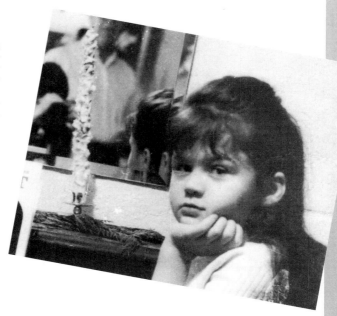

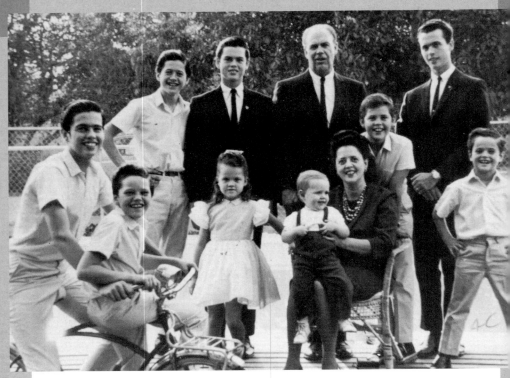

The whole family—looks like I forgot to smile. (*Osmond Family Archive*)

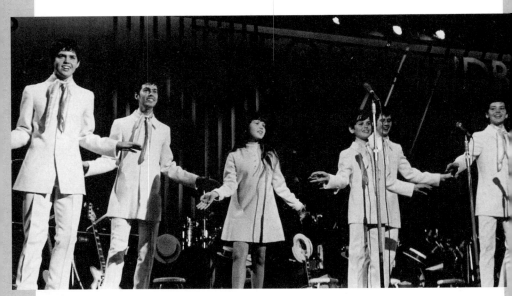

On stage, front and center, with no place to hide. (*Osmond Family Archive*)

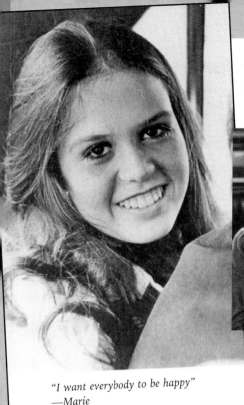

This photo was for my fans . . . making others happy was my career goal. (*Osmond Family Archive photo by Virl Osmond*)

"I want everybody to be happy"
—Marie

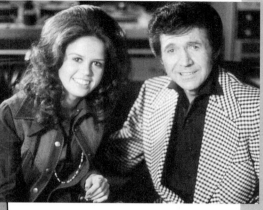

Sonny James, me, and my hair in the recording studio. I was thirteen when he produced my first record *Paper Roses*. (*Osmond Family Archive*)

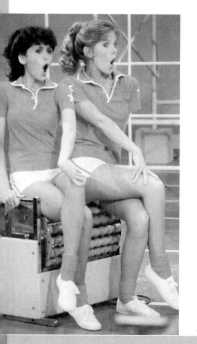

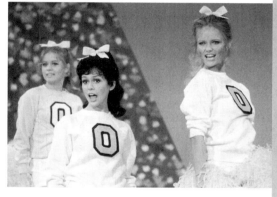

Cheryl Tiegs and I doing a cheer . . . I felt constantly surrounded by gorgeous girls. (*Osmond Family Archive*)

Debby Boone and I on the original show. She had the hit song "You Light Up My Life." My life at that time was focused on trying to lighten my waistline. (*Osmond Family Archive*)

I made my debut at age three with Andy Williams. He's been a great friend to all of the Osmonds over the years. (*Osmond Family Archive*)

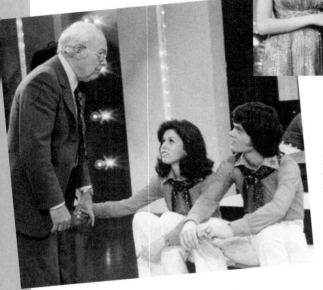

Father was usually on hand with advice and an encouraging word. (*Osmond Family Archive*)

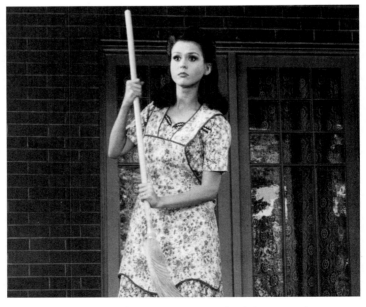

Portraying my mother in a 1982 television movie, *Side by Side*. Talk about looking like a Stepford wife! (*Osmond Family Archive*)

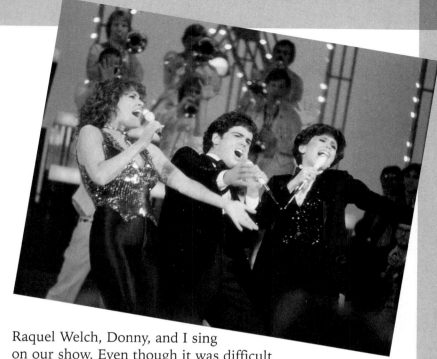

Raquel Welch, Donny, and I sing
on our show. Even though it was difficult
for me to stand next to the beauties of the 70s,
Donny loved it! (*Osmond Family Archive*)

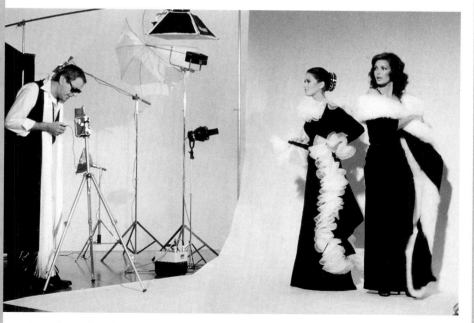

Another slender star of the 70s . . . Jaclyn Smith has those great
cheekbones. I've always had to paint mine on. (*Osmond Family
Archive*)

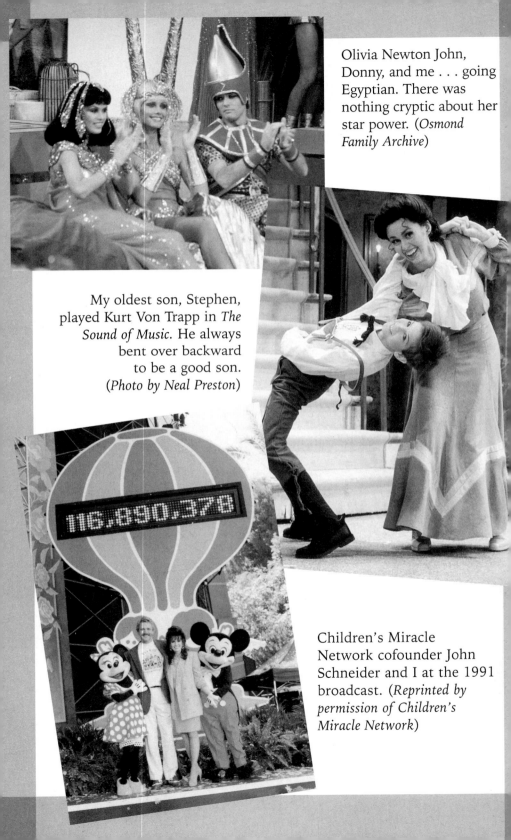

Olivia Newton John, Donny, and me . . . going Egyptian. There was nothing cryptic about her star power. (*Osmond Family Archive*)

My oldest son, Stephen, played Kurt Von Trapp in *The Sound of Music*. He always bent over backward to be a good son. (*Photo by Neal Preston*)

Children's Miracle Network cofounder John Schneider and I at the 1991 broadcast. (*Reprinted by permission of Children's Miracle Network*)

I've carried on my mother's tradition of making everyone matching Christmas pj's. Stephen, Jessica, and Rachael . . . this was (gasp) ten years ago. (*Osmond Family Archive*)

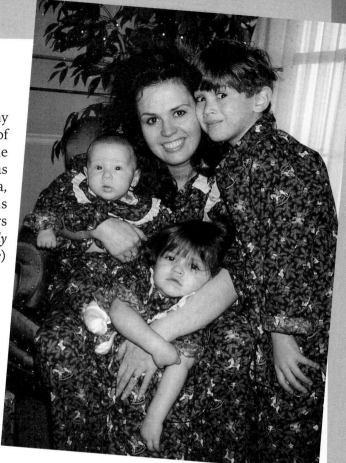

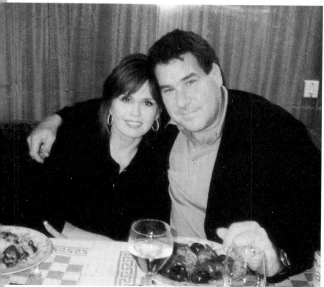

Brian—my husband and friend. (*Osmond Family Archive*)

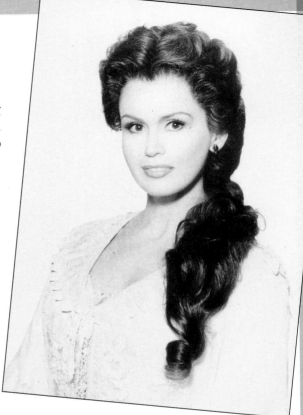

As "Anna" in *The King and I* in 1997. (*Photo by Eduardo Patino*)

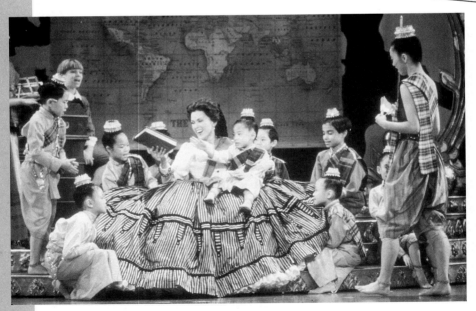

On stage with the *King and I* children—aren't they cute? (*Photo by Joan Marcus*)

years, this has become like a ceremony for me because I know that when I return home, I will have a precious baby wearing this outfit. I couldn't wait to see Matthew dressed in it, but somehow, as I was packing it, I felt that wasn't going to happen as I had planned. I couldn't say why. It was just one of those prevailing feelings, like when you try on a white sweater in the store and you get a vision of salad dressing down the front of it, or a kid sneezing cherry Popsicle near you the first time you wear it. As a second thought, I threw a little hand-me-down nightie that had been worn by my three-year-old, Brandon, into my suitcase too. I remember shaking off the premonition as a silly worry. After all, what could go wrong with infant wear? There are no zippers, no buttons, no hemlines, no cuffs; I mean, it's pretty much a sack, tied at the bottom.

Sure enough, the little homecoming outfit looked adorable on Matthew—for all of five minutes. I dressed him, wrapped him in his blanket, and put him in the bassinet in my hospital room while I finished packing.

Just as I was closing my suitcase, a noise came from the bassinet. It was the unmistakable sound of an infant expelling seven pounds of "stuff" from an eight-pound body. Not only was there spit-up from his face to his waist, but the other end had done its job from his tush to his toes, through the diaper, the outfit, the satin receiving blanket, and even the bassinet sheets. It was one of those times when baby wipes are as useless as Kleenex on an oil spill. I had to strip him down, give him a sponge bath, rinse out the clothes and blanket, and start from scratch.

I dug the little hand-me-down nightie out of the bottom of my suitcase. I didn't have an extra blanket. One of the nurses insisted I borrow an undershirt and baby blanket from the nursery. They were stamped with the name of the hospital, like little regulation prison wear. I should have had her take a mug shot of Matthew before his escape. When he is older and wants to see his presentation outfit, he'll have to visit the hospital where he busted out.

I can laugh about this now, but I remember feeling upset about my baby's having to wear the old nightie home and be swaddled in a hospital blanket. I told myself that I was over-reacting, that it was only an outfit. Besides, who was going to see him? It was three o'clock in the morning.

I knew it was a bigger issue than a ruined baby blanket. With six kids you start managing everything a body can ex-pel with a shrug and a wet washcloth. It was more about my feelings of not being ready to go home from the hospital. I wanted it to be a memorable occasion, especially knowing I would probably never again give birth. I knew I was com-pleting a season of my life. I needed time to pause and recognize that passage, which from my first child to my last had spanned seventeen years. I wanted it to be more ceremonious and special. Instead, I felt as if I had been given a pat on the back and told, "Good job in the service of procreation. Now pick up your childbearing honors and get on with it."

Pregnancy and childbirth are not illnesses, but I think our current system of discharging a new mother from the hospital so soon after giving birth is full of hazard. It may save money overall, but I have to question what the cost is to a woman's well-being and the welfare of her infant. They are sending home an exhausted, hormonally confused, phys-ically stressed woman with a tiny, fragile being who needs twenty-four-hour care. I think that alone is enough to cause depression in almost anyone.

It seems even more absurd when you consider that pro football players get more time off to recover after a game than many women get after delivering a baby the size of a football out of their bodies.

Women of my mother's generation usually had a hospital stay of five to seven full days following the birth of a baby. This gave them time to recover, get much-needed rest, and learn about caring for their infants without worrying about meals, housework, and other children. It also gave new mothers the chance to talk over their concerns with a supportive nursing staff that could dispel fears and teach them confidence before they had to handle child care on their own. Despite my feelings, staying at the hospital was not an option I could consider. I had six others at home who missed and needed their mother.

✦

The only people who knew of my plan were Brian, the doctor, and the late-night nurses, who invited me to the chocolate party they were holding at the nurses' station at three A.M. So that's how they stay alert all night long . . . brownie buzz. They had planned a clean getaway for me. They plotted out a course through the hallways to the service elevator, then down to the back entrance of the hospital, where I could sneak out. I gave all of my bouquets of flowers to the staff, along with many hugs and thank-yous. I wrapped a sweater around my shoulders and pulled the receiving blanket up to cover my baby's face. Brian pushed me in a wheelchair as the hospital staff scouted the hallways ahead to make sure they were clear and then waved us on. The last turn took us through the geriatric ward and out of the building. It didn't escape my thoughts that I was bringing a new life out into the world through a door others entered near the conclusion of theirs.

I gathered my suitcase and ducked quickly into the car while the paparazzi slept in nearby vans. Unnoticed, we drove off in the dark. Little did I know then how much darker it was going to get.

8

<hr>

Someone to Watch Over Me

I want my mother.

On the drive home from the hospital, I couldn't help but remember my first day home after the last time I gave birth. My mother was waiting there for me. She took the baby from my arms and said, "You need to go upstairs and get in bed. I'll fix you something to eat."

When I protested, telling her I was fine, she just said, "Now you mind me. Get in bed. Go on. I'm more stubborn than you."

It didn't matter that I was thirty years old, she was my mother and she was deciding what was best for me. My other kids were content and happy to be with Grandma, so I went to bed as my mother ordered. The feeling of being looked after and having her make household decisions was so comforting that I started to cry. Even when she brought me up a tray with a dinner plate full of mashed potatoes, sweet peas, and roast beef, I was still weeping with happiness: sitting in bed, eating green peas, and sobbing, simply because it was so wonderful to have my mother near me. I know I was having signs of the baby blues, but it was okay because she was there.

That was ten years ago. As much as my mother would have loved to help with this baby, she had suffered a series of minor strokes and a broken back in recent years. She has had to slow down a bit, though I have to tell you, my mother's "slowed down" is everyone else's average pace. She was still active, but she had been advised by doctors to not lift or carry anything, which was impossible to avoid in my household with three children under age three.

◆

Around the holidays, when every airplane is full to capacity of people going wherever they call home, I feel a sense of melancholy at how many people live away from their families. Family is everything to me. It's important to me that my children be around other family members, and especially that they know their grandparents. I loved my grandparents, and Brian was very fond of his too. I gained a deep sense of personal worth from my grandmothers. They taught me things a mother can't always teach a stubborn teenager, like the joys of charity work, house-cleaning tips, a coveted custard recipe, and more. I loved working side by side with them, learning through example how to make jam, can fresh fruit, lift a stain, prune a hedge, and even catch a fish and clean and prepare it. Most of all, they made me understand that it's better to collect stories of our heritage through spending time together than it is to accumulate things that will tarnish and fade.

I know their grandparents can talk about and teach my children about life in ways I never could. They have a wisdom that has been gathered over time. My mother is a teacher, businesswoman, computer fanatic, and chronicler of our genealogy. My father is a great craftsman, people person, and storyteller. His singing voice is beautiful, and his artistic talent is such that he has helped me sculpt a doll or two for my porcelain doll business I started ten years ago. Besides their individual talents, they have a knack, when they are with my children, for slipping a piece of knowledge in with a fun activity. They do it for the kids' benefit, but I still learn something new every time my parents are around.

During one of my mother's visits, I came home from work to find the house filled with the unmistakable aroma of her fresh-baked bread. I tossed my briefcase on the stairs by the entryway. I couldn't wait to cut a thick slice and slather it with butter.

I was greeted at the kitchen door by my kids, who had flour covering their hands and faces. I could tell they were having a great afternoon with Grandma, learning baking lessons, which double as life lessons . . . gently kneading dough and giving it time to rise, just as she taught me when I was a little girl. I was pretty sure the bread would still be warm because I could feel the heat from the oven.

"It smells fantastic," I said to my mother, hugging her while at the same time scouting out the fresh-baked loaves. Where were they?

My mother shook her head. "Take a good long whiff," she advised, laughing, "because the scent is all that's left."

I turned to look at my kids, licking the last traces of butter off their fingers. Rachael shrugged and said, "Sorry, Mom. We didn't know you'd be home this early. You can hang out with Grandma now. There's a bunch of baking pans that need washing, and you always say that doing dishes is good conversation time. See ya."

My mother will often tell me something, usually just matter-of-factly and in passing, that I find to be amazingly profound. Recently she was describing a time when my older brothers were little boys and she was standing nearby watching them play with Tinker Toys and Lincoln Logs (the Legos of the sixties) on the floor, and helping them fit the pieces together periodically.

"I was thinking, Marie," my mother recalled, "that this must be what our Father in heaven does too. He stands over us, watching us busy ourselves with our own creations. He doesn't interfere, knowing our happiness comes from making our lives the way we want them to be. But I'm sure He'd love it if we'd look up once in a while and ask for directions."

◆

As we pulled into the driveway with Matthew long before dawn, I knew I had to put aside my memories of my mother's excellent care. I had seven children who wanted their mother, and I needed to take care of them.

After I changed the baby and got him settled in his bassinet, I went around to the beds of each of my sleeping children. I cuddled and rocked my toddlers. There is no such thing as the terrible twos when they're sleeping. That's the time you truly see and appreciate exactly what they are: little angels. The horns don't usually sprout out of their heads until after breakfast, and they hide their three-pronged forks until just before naptime.

I kissed each of the older kids and whispered, "Mom's home," checked to make sure no one had acquired a tattoo in my absence, and then I crawled in bed and fell into a restless sleep. As any mother knows, once you have children you rarely experience a true deep sleep. You become aware of every creak of the floorboards, every cough, sneeze, and whimper. Sometimes the one whimpering is you, but that's easy enough to ignore because, as any mother will tell you, you don't have time for that.

Later the next day, Brian left for Los Angeles to finalize the closing on the new house. We were supposed to have moved out of the house we had been renting by July 1, and the owners were charging an outrageous amount of money for every day past that deadline. Though it bothered me that he was leaving, Brian was anxious that we were throwing so much money away on a house we no longer occupied. He was determined to get our belongings out of there and turn over the keys. The new house had been occupied by a family who had pets, so I wanted to have the carpets professionally cleaned before we moved in. I knew all of this had to be done before we could return to L.A., but having Brian leave so soon after the birth was hard on me emotionally. I wanted him to share the first few days of the baby's life with me so badly that I felt sullen and tearful. I was grieving a passing era in my life. My childbearing years had come to an end. Matthew would be my "Omega" child. Brian and I chalked up my emotional state to the baby blues. The amount of time left to get everything squared away in L.A. was dwindling, and now that the baby had safely arrived, it seemed practical to finish the move as soon as possible.

Knowing that Matthew was the last baby I would give birth to made me want to take notice of everything about him. I wanted to stop time for a while, to pack away the reality of my schedule and just be with him. They are little for such a short time, and in those first months they change by the day. Every mother knows those adoring looks they give you, those brief months when you are their whole world and that end precisely the minute they learn to say the word *no*. So you gotta get it when you can.

But I think for Brian, the next important thing on his list after the birth of his son was getting the L.A. house transaction settled.

There wasn't a way for me to ask him to stay. It didn't make sense for him to stay. But feelings don't always make sense. Feelings don't pay attention to a schedule, a deadline, or even a reasonable request. Sometimes I look at the passion with which my younger children will express their feelings. All emotions, from complete joy to deep hurt to fear or anger, come out of them with unabashed ease. Sorrow in a two-year-old child comes out as streams of tears, red-faced wails, and curling up on the floor. Usually, that total expression of feeling is somewhat buried and put under control by the time we reach school age, but I don't think the intensity of the feeling itself ever really changes. At my most vulnerable times as an adult, I can still feel the heightened emotions that I did as a little girl. I was full of sorrow that Brian was leaving. I wanted to wail and curl up on the bed. I felt completely abandoned. I was still weak and tired from giving birth and I wanted to be protected from the outside. Nothing seemed as important to me. Not the show, not the moving, not any work deadlines. I felt it should all come second for Brian too, behind being with me and enjoying the new baby.

I once heard a metaphor about the differences between men and women that made sense to me. Men were compared to mountains, sturdy and solid, looking at life as something to conquer. They compartmentalize and work from a list of priorities. Women are more like rivers. We go with the landscape, turning and bending to get over the rough spots. We move around or through whatever stands in our way to keep things flowing. We stay open to change and work on what's most important at that moment.

◆

B rian arranged to have my girlfriend Patty fly in from L.A. to spend a couple of days with me. Patty has a comforting way of taking care of situations and an extraordinary talent for making everything run smoothly. She's the administrator of Larry King's office. With his CNN interviews with celebrities and politicians, his charity work, and his speaking engagements, Larry's schedule is incredibly complex. Patty and Larry are such attention-to-details people that together they could set the time on the Universal Time Clock. I've known her most of my life, since I was ten and she was eleven. (Yeah, Patty, you're always gonna be older than I am.) She was one of the first girls I ever trusted. While I was growing up, my experience with girls who sought out my friendship usually proved to be disappointing. They would come over pretending to want to hang out with me and then spend all their time trying to get the attention of one of my brothers.

Patty was different. We hit it off right away. She and I still have an inexplicable connection. On my worst days, I'll get a phone message from Patty saying, "Hey, nerd!" (Isn't she sweet?) "What's going on? I can feel you aren't happy. Call me." I have the same intuition about her. I'll call from out of the country, sometimes just waking up in the middle of the night feeling that something's wrong in Patty's life. She'll have been right in the middle of a hardship and say, "I can't believe you are calling right now. You won't believe what is going on. What time is it in London, anyway?"

She is also a person I can count on to be brutally honest. Sometimes it's startling, but I usually find it refreshing and can laugh about it later. For example, if I say, "Oh, I feel so puffy and out of shape today," most of my friends might say something like, "Don't think about it. You look great."

Not Patty. Patty will say, "You should. Your arms are flabby and your butt is getting wide." I learned quickly not to ask Patty's opinion right before I go on stage. Otherwise, I would be interviewing Kevin Bacon or Ted Danson and thinking, "Hmm. I hope this outfit covers my flabby arms."

It's impossible for Patty to just hang out. If she's at my house, she has to be active. I'll take a five-minute phone call and come back to find that she's alphabetized my pantry, swept and mopped the floors, and made a handy homework checklist for the kids to hang on the freshly polished refrigerator door. My kids adore her because she can make the most complicated sibling squabble seem as if it has a quick solution when she quips, "Get over it!" The kids usually giggle and forget what they were fighting about in the first place.

So Patty arrived at the airport just as Brian was leaving and did what she does so well. She got the baby clothes in order, threw laundry in, and tried to keep the noise level to a minimum so I could rest. She answered the phone and the door, and controlled the length of time visitors stayed. Let me tell you something: Judge Judy has nothing on Patty. She'll tell you exactly who, what, where, when, and why. And if you don't listen to her, she'll toss her head with a "don't come crying to me" attitude. I hope everyone has a friend like Patty. Oh, they can drive you crazy, but you can't help but be crazy about them when you know they do it all out of great loyalty and love. I was so grateful to have her there, even if it was only for a couple of days. I knew she had to get back to her job, but as soon as she was gone it became apparent that disorganization was going to rule. If I had any thoughts of avoiding my routine for a couple more days, that hope was being squashed before my eyes. My routine was already begging for attention every five minutes.

The phone rang continuously with calls about business decisions that I had to make. Can you do a photo shoot? Meet with a new publicist? Do a doll signing in Las Vegas? Rehearse music for the Miss America pageant? Do an interview with *McCall's* magazine? How soon can you be ready to go? Two weeks? One week? Three days? Tomorrow? In fact, are you busy right now?

The doorbell seemed to be ringing even more now that Patty was gone. So many of my friends in Utah wanted to see the baby. Women from the church, whom I love, brought by casseroles and baked goods for the family so I didn't have to cook. The kids' cousins and friends came over to play and ended up staying for sleepovers.

My two nannies, Jill and Melissa, would come over in the morning to take the kids to the pool, the park, or the movies. One of them would usually watch the older kids and the other the two toddlers. While I feel blessed to be in a position where I can bring in outside help and have been fortunate to have phenomenal people around my children, emotionally I still missed the security of having my mother or another family member who could help direct traffic and make decisions in those early weeks after the birth. They don't have to ask what needs to be done or ask permission. They just clear the path and make things happen because they love you.

My grandmother Osmond used to tell me when I was younger, "You need to take care of yourself, Marie, because no one else is going to." I questioned at the time why she would tell me that. I thought it sounded selfish, that it meant you should always think of yourself first. But when I learned of her history and what she had had to do to survive, I knew she hadn't had any options. She had no one else to take care of her.

Her husband, my grandfather, died young from a damaged liver after being kicked by a horse. She was widowed with three little boys, two of whom were preschool aged and one of whom (my father) was only two weeks old. She had to support herself and her babies, so she went to work in the fields, cutting grain with a machete. She couldn't carry the children into the field with her, so she would tether the two older ones to a tree with leashes wrapped around their waists and put the baby in a wooden box, which served as a bassinet. Working in the fields, she saved enough money to open and run a boardinghouse, which allowed her to be near her children.

Whenever I think about my life as being difficult or stressful, I remember Grandma Osmond. I think of her life, her determination to provide for her family, and her will to get by on her own. I have more understanding of her wise words now. Sorry it took so long to sink in, Grandma! She was one tough lady. I like to think that I'm from her sturdy stock and have the genes to be one tough lady too.

Like my grandmother, I'm not a person who is afraid of hard work or of taking a plunge into a new venture. The difference was I didn't take care of myself. I've been in the entertainment business since I was three years old, when I first appeared on *The Andy Williams Show*. I've been "busy" for thirty-eight of my forty-one years. I've accomplished most things in my life through sheer determination. I really don't think I have as much talent as I have drive, but one of my greatest fears is that I might waste a talent that I have been given. My life has always been busy and hectic because I wanted it to be that way. (I've never come up short on having the drive to get done what was needed, but it took postpartum depression for me to learn to put it in park for a while, to actually see what I really wanted.)

Just like our babies, we all learn to say no early on, but it seems to be a word that many women forget too easily. I think in my case, I don't say it because I don't want to seem uncaring. In my mind, taking care of myself by saying no to a request means that someone else might have to go without.

The only person I was really good at saying no to was myself. "No, you shouldn't sleep when the house is messy." "No, you shouldn't eat so much or you'll never lose weight for the show." "No, you can't rest when there are so many people who need you." "No, you can't let yourself be sad." "There's no time for tears. No. Get over it!"

On my third day at home, I was up early to feed the baby. I started to look at what kind of shape the house was really in and what we needed to pack and move from the house in Utah to our new home in L.A. I was anxious, so busying myself seemed like a good idea. I think many women are good at busying themselves as a way to hide pain. I found some cardboard boxes and started sorting out toys and towels, summer wear from winter wear, thinking that I would pack while the baby slept. I felt I was getting something accomplished, and it distracted me from the gloom that seemed to be creeping into my heart. By the end of the afternoon, I was exhausted and very weepy. I knew I should lie down for a while, thinking that if I took one of my "crisis naps," as I've always called them, I'd be okay in an hour.

While doing the original *Donny & Marie* show, as well as during years of touring, I grew quite adept at crisis napping, which meant grabbing twenty or thirty minutes of sleep wherever and whenever I could. I would curl up on the floor under the makeup table in my dressing room and take a quick nap while they changed the set. I could sit on an instrument case backstage, lean my head against the curtains, and doze off. I've been known to grab a corner of carpet in an airport, a photographer's studio, or a soundstage and fall fast asleep for however long I had before the next thing on the schedule. My body became so conditioned to sleeping in this manner that it still has an internal alarm set to wake me every hour to make sure everything is going along on time.

The nannies, trying to be considerate, told me they were going to pack up the kids, take them to the pool for a swim, and get them dinner at the snack shack so I could have time to myself. I couldn't tell them the truth: that the last thing I really wanted was to be alone. I wanted to be surrounded by love and nurtured back to health. I wanted someone to watch over me.

When the baby woke me up an hour later, I was famished. I knew that I was not getting proper nourishment, which meant my baby wasn't either, considering that I was nursing. The kitchen was understocked, to say the least, because the house had been unoccupied for most of the year. The kids had been eating casseroles and other food brought by the women from our church and getting fast food when they were out for the day.

Feeling shaky, I went downstairs to see what I could find to eat. The refrigerator was empty except for milk and juice. The cabinets just held cereal and some canned goods. It crossed my mind to order from a restaurant and have it delivered, but I knew that would take some time, and I was beyond hungry. It seemed the effort it would take to order food was more than I could muster. I also didn't want to open the front door for a delivery person, because the paparazzi, having missed their photo opportunity at the hospital, had taken to circling my neighborhood, waiting for me to make an appearance. I was trapped in my own house, alone with a newborn baby. Looking back, I know I could have made a phone call to any number of friends or family members who would have dropped what they were doing and brought over groceries, but I couldn't let myself ask for help. In my mind, it really didn't feel like an option. Again, I said no to myself. I was thinking, "No, Marie. Don't bother anyone. They have enough problems of their own. They don't need to take care of you. You can get by on your own."

I opened one more cabinet and found a jar of peanut butter. No crackers or bread, just peanut butter. I got out a spoon and dug in. My head was pounding from being hungry, my body was sore, and my spine felt as if it could splinter from overuse. The doctor had warned me to go easy and not to lift or go up and down the stairs too often, but I thought his advice was for somebody else. It couldn't be for anyone as tough as me. I could handle it. I could have a baby and get right back to work. I could get my family moved, make business decisions, get back in shape. I could get past the baby blues. I could do whatever needed to be done.

Five minutes later, I was sitting on the kitchen floor, heaving with sobs, and all I could think was, "This can't possibly be me." This couldn't be me, collapsed in hysteria, not even recognizing my own wails. This was not me, shaken to the core, sliding into a despair of the deepest kind. Whoever this was, she had no control of her emotions. Whoever this was, I wanted nothing to do with her. I wanted her away from my house, my children, and my baby. Whoever this was, I could tell she was falling over the edge. I tried to back away from the cliff, but she had a firm hold on me. I could feel myself slipping and desperately tried to hang on, my fingers dug into the very foundation of the life I had structured: wife, mother, entertainer, and businesswoman. But I couldn't climb back out and she couldn't save herself. My grip gave way and she took me down with her.

9

What a Pain in the Neck!

I'm in a semidrugged state of consciousness in the basement of my neighbor's house. I can't think of anywhere I'd rather be. It's dark, cool, and quiet, and I feel as though I could stay down here forever. I'm not sure how much time has passed, but my energy level isn't enough for me to climb the stairs and join the life going on upstairs. My exhausted body holds me hostage in this bed, and I stay willingly. I feel peaceful and secure. I want to sleep for a year. Just two days ago I thought I couldn't get any lower than sitting on the floor, crying, eating peanut butter, but now, here I am in a basement.

◆

My descent to the basement began when the wrecking ball that demolished my emotional well-being in the kitchen came to rest on my shoulder and neck, manifesting as physical pain. I felt like a female Atlas, carrying the weight of the world on my shoulders.

It started in my first week home from the hospital as a stiff neck, which I attributed to sleeping with the baby cuddled against my arm. Halfway through the day, the tautness of my muscles felt like a clamp on my shoulder.

My daughter Brianna, who was only twenty months old, was having a hard time adjusting to a new little one taking up my attention. She was feeling displaced and wanted to be held by me as much as possible. By late afternoon, trying to lift her sent a stabbing pain through my ribs, my shoulder, and up my neck.

That night when I put the kids to bed, I could no longer turn my head, and I could barely bend over to kiss them good-night. I had taken the pain reliever the doctor gave me at the hospital, but it wasn't helping at all. The baby was fussy and irritable, and I was afraid he was picking up on my stressed state of body and mind. I was not producing enough milk to meet his nutritional needs, so I started supplementing his feedings with formula. I had hoped that I would be able to nurse until I started back to work. Putting him on a bottle so soon made me feel I was failing him miserably. I wanted his first week of life to be so peaceful; instead it was full to the brim with ringing phones, streams of strangers, and a mother who couldn't seem to stop crying.

After he fell asleep, I thought I could ease my tense muscles by taking a hot shower. By this time my neck was throbbing so badly that I just stood under the hot water and leaned against the wall for what seemed like forever. I pressed my hands against the tile and began to sob. I tried to shake off the emotion, but the effort only resulted in more tears. No amount of tears seemed to relieve the emotional pain I felt, and the hot shower did not improve my neck pain at all. I couldn't even raise my arm high enough to towel off my hair and face. I tried to lie down and relax, but the muscles in my neck and shoulder had started to spasm to the point that I couldn't even catch my breath. After an hour, I started to feel panicked about not being able to move or breathe easily. I pulled the phone off the bedside stand and onto the pillow next to my head and called Brian in Los Angeles.

"Brian, I'm in so much pain." I was gasping by this time. "What should I do?"

He thought I should call an ambulance, but I said no, it would scare the kids. Then he suggested that he call our neighbors, LuAnn and Mike. I looked at the clock and, realizing it was one in the morning, said, "No, Brian. I don't want to bother them in the middle of the night. I'll be okay."

I don't really know what I expected him to do from Los Angeles, but I desperately needed to connect with him because I was feeling so much pain and so alone.

We had been close friends with LuAnn and Mike for over ten years. We'd shared vacations, and our children had always been playmates. Her teenage daughters baby-sat my younger kids and helped me around the house. They lived in the house directly behind ours, and our friendship was so strong that we had a gate installed in the backyard fence between our properties so we could cross back and forth without going around the block.

Shortly after Brian and I hung up, it was obvious he had ignored my request not to call them. Mike appeared at the back door, his face full of concern. When he saw that I couldn't move my head or even stand up to talk to him, he told me he was taking me to the emergency room. I leaned against the door and said, "No Mike, that's not necessary. It's late."

"How do you know this isn't meningitis?" he asked. "I'm calling LuAnn."

In a matter of minutes, LuAnn was there to help me get dressed and into the car. Tears were running down my face from trying to get my arm into the sleeve of my dress. LuAnn had called the baby-sitters, who were staying at a nearby apartment, and had them come over to stay at the house with the kids. I was still protesting the need to go to the hospital, but LuAnn insisted.

"This is not right, Marie," she told me. "You shouldn't be in this much pain after having a baby. We're not leaving you here. We're going to the hospital."

Lu, as I call her, is one of the sweetest women walking the earth. She is gentle, soft-spoken, and filled with grace, but she is also strong and determined. So if she is ever insistent, she means business, and nothing can change her mind. I love her for it.

The doctor who had delivered Matthew happened to be at the hospital that night and was called down to the emergency room to check on me. He couldn't believe that I was in that much pain postdelivery. He thought I might have done damage to my back and ordered an injection of a muscle relaxant. That shot relieved only about 25 percent of the pain. When he came back to check on me, he was amazed that I was still in major discomfort from muscle spasm.

"I have a pretty high pain tolerance," I said. "So if I'm here, it means it's not just a cramp. Bring on the big-boy stuff!"

He was laughing, maybe at me, but I figured if I had come to the emergency room, I was not leaving without relief! The second shot took me to another level of existence altogether, and I remember lying there thinking, "Good thing I don't have to drive myself home." Remember how bad I am at directions? In this state of "lala" I would probably have had to read the car manual to figure out how to put the key in the ignition.

One of the nurses on duty that night gave me a poem that he had obviously photocopied many times. It started out with lines like "Imagine you are sitting by a babbling brook, the birds are singing, the sun is warm . . ." I stopped reading after the third line. I couldn't imagine the babbling brook. I couldn't even imagine why I would want to finish that stupid poem. The nurse was standing nearby and encouraged me to keep reading.

"Great," I thought. "I can't even escape the pressure of letting down a nurse by not reading his poem." I continued reading for his sake and then I started cracking up laughing. Three more lines down the page the poem read something like: "Imagine the person who caused you stress. You can see his face in the water . . . because you're holding his head under the surface. Now, just let him up for one quick breath, and then back under. Feel better?"

He gave me a copy of the poem, and we even ran it one day on *Donny & Marie.* It was a great stress buster, and I carried it in my wallet for at least four months.

The doctor gave me a prescription painkiller and a stern warning to take my life down ten notches for at least a week before I did permanent muscle damage.

On the way home, I was feeling groggy but so much better that I was almost happy. I thanked my friends and apologized for getting them up in the middle of the night. LuAnn swung around in the front seat to face me and said, "Oh, don't think you're going home. I'm not leaving you there with seven kids. You're staying with us."

I told her I was sure I would be okay now, but Lu was hearing none of it. And really, what was my choice right then? To open the passenger door, leap out, and roll down the median strip?

My mother, in another of her moments of wisdom, once told me, "You have to be as gracious in the receiving as you are in the giving. If you're not, you deny the other person the blessing of giving." I knew this was true in Lu's case. If people are blessed for giving, then this woman is the Bill Gates of blessings. She was determined to ease my worries, and I'll always be grateful for the way she and her husband stepped in to rescue me in my deep need that night.

Mike and Lu had remodeled their basement into a lovely guest room, with a cozy bed and a comfortable atmosphere. It was quiet and private, the perfect place to recover. Lu got me settled in the room and then went to my house to explain to the baby-sitters what was going on and ask them to stay on with the kids. She arranged for them to be with the children for the next day and night, and then gathered up supplies for Matthew and brought him home with her. Just knowing that Lu was taking care of my baby and that my other children would be looked after gave me a great sense of peace. I crawled under the quilt and drifted off into the deepest sleep that is possible for me.

I have no idea how many hours I slept, but the next thing I knew, Lu was bringing me a breakfast tray. She was worried that I hadn't eaten for so long. She brought the baby downstairs for me to feed and cuddle. As comforting as it was to be taken care of, my heart was heavy. I was repeatedly sending myself the message: What's wrong with you? Get up. Go home. Be with your children.

I was so sad, and I told Lu that I should get back home.

"Absolutely not," she said. "You can barely hold your eyes open right now. Everyone is fine. I love having this time to bond with Matthew, and my daughters are thrilled about having a baby here. I've been over to check on the other children and they're good. They'll come see you later today. You have to rest."

And rest is what I did. I don't think I was awake for more than sixty minutes over the next twenty-four hours. I would get up and go upstairs, and then fall asleep sitting up after fifteen minutes. I'm sure some of it was the prescription painkillers making me drowsy, but I was still so exhausted. Lu would make me something to eat, I would see the kids for a couple of minutes, and then I would feel as if I were going to collapse. My body insisted that I give in, and my mind lost the battle.

Brian had been calling and getting updates from Mike, and I guess after the third call Lu asked Mike to tell Brian to come home. She said that even though I was getting better physically, I needed his emotional support, and it would help me for him to be there. He caught the next plane out of Los Angeles.

Back in Utah, he came downstairs to see me. He wanted me to come home with him, but I was very weepy and didn't want the kids to see me this shaken. I couldn't communicate to him my feelings of loneliness and my inability to completely cope in this emotional state. I could feel myself shutting down, protecting my heart, because I felt he was unable to perceive how much I needed his full support. Instead, I withdrew, saying I could handle it.

Lu said that I should stay awhile longer. Brian agreed and went to talk to the kids. We all thought I was having a reaction to overdoing and would be back to myself soon.

That evening I felt so much better that I got dressed and went upstairs. I suggested that Brian and I take Lu and Mike to a restaurant for dinner as a way to thank them for taking care of me. I thought getting out for a little while would be good. I called Brian on his cell phone, and he said he would meet us. One hour passed, then two, and I started getting tired again. I wasn't sure where Brian was, but I didn't want to wait anymore. Mike finally ran to a restaurant and picked up a carryout order, and we ate dinner around Lu's dining table.

Finally, Brian arrived, excusing himself for being late. He had been caught up on the phone rescheduling studio time with musicians so he could be there with me. I didn't really expect that he should put his work on hold, but once again,

I felt he was unable to see that I needed assurance that everything would be okay and that he was there to take over.

Brian had called my parents to tell them where I was and what was going on, so the next morning they drove down to visit. The nannies, Jill and Melissa, brought the other children over, and we had a little family gathering. I told my mother and Lu that I couldn't remember the last time I had slept for as many hours as I had the past two nights. But even though I felt rested, I was still really weepy and shaky. I could tell that my parents were concerned about my mental state, so I struggled to pull myself together and put on "the smile." I didn't want them to worry. Brian thought it was time that I came home. I knew the kids missed me. My neck and shoulder pain had become bearable, so I went downstairs to gather my things.

Lu followed me downstairs and said, "I really don't want to send you back home yet to that house full of kids. I think you need more time to rest."

On the inside I was in turmoil. I wanted to stay too. But I couldn't just drop out of my life. I had a husband and children to care for, a move to make, weight to lose, calls to return, doll signings to appear at, and a national television show to host in a matter of weeks. The clock was running, and there was no chance of signaling a time-out. I had to get up off the bench, leave the haven of this basement, and jump back into action. So I put on my game face, hugged Lu, and said, "I'm so much better. Really. I'm ready to take over."

I left knowing that my words had not completely convinced Lu, and to be honest, I believed them even less.

10

◆

Highway Hypnosis: You're Getting Very Shaky

The car I drive every day seats eight people. Eight! Most of the time, all the seats are full. There's the "baby" row, which has three car seats strapped in directly behind the driver. Many pacifiers have been lost between them, collecting with all forms of goop in those hard-to-reach spaces. I've tried to retrieve one or two. It's as impossible as those arcade games at the grocery store in which the goal is to get the crane claws around a stuffed toy and lift it. You may be able to reach between the car seats and hook a pacifier, but it's sure to drop from your fingers before you get it to the surface.

The child that rides "shotgun" has the best seat (control of the tunes), and the bidding for that seat usually begins hours before we leave the house. "I call front seat," one of the kids will shout out. "I called it before breakfast," another will claim. Usually the winner comes up with something like, "I called it before you were even born!" I try to stay out of it because otherwise, to keep any peace, I would have to pull over every three-quarters of a mile and rotate them. Once the front seat is taken, the others are filled in by priority, windows taken first, with a sleepover friend or two thrown in the center seats. All my "frequent riders" know that "good behavior may be redeemed for a seating upgrade."

I know many moms who dread car trips with children, but I actually find them comforting. It's the only time I have every kid in sight, present and accounted for. I love having my children near me, and being in the car can actually give me time to catch up on their lives without outside distraction. They seem to like it too. Brianna once pitched my ringing cell phone out the window at fifty-five miles per hour. She has to compete for my attention with six other kids, and she wasn't about to let an outside caller stand in her way.

And I wasn't about to let a bad case of baby blues stand in my way. I was pretty certain that the worst was behind me and I would feel like myself in a couple of days. After all, I'm a pretty positive person by nature. When faced with hardships in the past, I would maybe let myself cry one little tear, but then I would usually shake off the blues, pile the kids in the car to go get an ice cream, and mentally move on! So I was really tired of being blue this time, and I had already allowed myself one tear, or two, or twenty. Besides, twenty ice-cream cones in one sitting is too much for anyone. I get brain freeze around number fifteen, don't you?

I had planned to fly back to Los Angeles at the end of the week with all the kids and a baby-sitter. Brian had left Utah to go to San Francisco, where he was involved in producing a jazz album. I decided to switch my plans after I was warned that the tabloids had heard of my flight arrangements and were waiting at the airport to snap photos. I wasn't ready to face any photographers, tabloid or not, because I felt so out of shape and my face looked so puffy and tired. I made up my mind to drive back to L.A. with my kids. I felt as if I couldn't wait another day. I had to get the house in L.A. in order and get the children comfortable and ready for school before the second season of the show started. I found any decision making overwhelming at that time, even the no-brainers, so I was pleased I had made this one. No one else in my life seemed quite as pleased. They took turns trying to talk me out of it, saying, "Marie, you just gave birth two and a half weeks ago!" And "You're going to get too run down," and "What are you thinking?" I guess I wasn't thinking clearly, because it seemed I was hearing concern from everyone who knew of my decision to drive to L.A., especially from many of the friends who came to my baby shower the day of my planned departure.

My dear friends Lisa Hatch and Shawn King, along with Shawn's mother, Gerri Engemann, had arranged the baby shower for me. Poor Lisa had rescheduled the shower twice because of my going underground with neck and shoulder problems. She offered to cancel for the third time, saying, "I know you don't feel like yourself right now. We can do this later." But I knew how much trouble they had gone to in arranging it to cheer me up, and I wanted to see all my good friends in Utah before I went back to California.

What I mean is, I wanted to see them, but I really didn't want them to see me. My eyes were constantly swollen from sleepless nights, and worse, my kidneys appeared to be barely keeping up. My body was still retaining fluid, and I mean *fluid*. I sloshed when I walked!

Since I hadn't planned on giving birth in Utah, I only had maternity clothes with me. I wasn't about to wear a Pea in the Pod dress to the baby shower, especially since the pea was out of the pod, but I had no idea how to get to the mall without being caught by photographers. I called Lisa and asked her to please rescue me from a fashion faux pas, or, worse yet, rumors that I was in my fifth trimester because I was still wearing maternity dresses. She went to the mall with my charge card and found me something I could wear in public, but not without a play-by-play description of what a difficult task it was. At one point she jokingly called to say, "I'm in the WalMart lawn-and-garden department. They have some great pool covers we could sew some elastic into." She did end up finding me a dress, and I don't know anyone else who could have done that for me.

Lisa, my creative director and doll partner, is a great woman, a dedicated mom, an excellent businessperson, and one of the funniest women I know. We've lived through eleven babies and four husbands together. Enough said. She's been a true-blue friend, and believe me, she's seen me blue. She's even seen me without makeup. Lipstick too. (Don't tell my mother.) I've known her for almost seventeen years, and I hold our relationship dear.

Because we share a creative brain wave, when we're working on a new doll design, we shop at the same fabric store separately and, without talking, pick out identical fabric for the dress, the petticoats, and even the same lace trim and accessories for the hair. We've done this time and again. I can always trust her ideas to coincide exactly with how I envision designing the doll myself.

I knew that if Lisa, Shawn, and Gerri were in charge of the baby shower, it would be a beautiful event. It was. They had to hold it at a country club because the guest list had somehow exploded, but the one name that was missing was Shawn's. She had helped to plan the party, but because of my rescheduling, she was unable to attend. The room was sweetly decorated with table centerpieces, designed by Gerri, of stackable blocks and baby puzzle games and toys with bouquets of helium balloons attached. They were all for Matthew, with a note attached saying, "After six kids, we figured you needed to update the toy box."

What a bittersweet morning it was. I sat in the beautiful dress Lisa had picked out for me, surrounded by girlfriends who were there to show support and welcome my newborn. As much as I loved each of these women, I felt as if I were removed from the event, as if I were sitting in a dark movie theater, watching a screen full of light and fun, but just observing all of it. I felt almost robotic, putting on a show, trying to convince the group that everything was getting better.

I stood up to make a short thank-you speech and found my voice cracking with emotion four words into it. I explained that I was beating back the baby blues, that I was sure they understood, and told them that I appreciated their support. Even as I was saying those words, the painful reality struck me that what I was feeling was more than the baby blues. I had had the blues with my last birth. This was nothing like that experience. Something was very wrong with me. I'd always been able to rise to a social occasion, and this time I felt as if I were fading away minute by minute. I was being beaten back by something much larger than my own desire to respond to my friends.

After the shower, as we were packing the trunk of Lisa's car with the gifts I had received, it was all I could do to keep from hyperventilating. I was so anxious about all I had to do, and the hands on the clock seemed to be rotating faster and faster, along with my breathing. My thoughts crashed against one another inside of my head: "I can't keep up. Don't you dare fall apart. You're weak. I have to pull myself together."

Another friend of mine, Linda Glather, followed Lisa and me back to the house after the shower. She helped us get the gifts into the house and then was supposed to leave with Lisa but didn't. I was standing, looking around at the house with my mouth open, I'm sure. Being in the controlled environment of the beautifully decorated country club made me see in spectravision exactly how disorderly my house had become since the baby was born. Suitcases were half packed, kids' toys were scattered on the floor, laundry was spilling out of the dryer, and the kitchen counter was covered with unwashed dishes. With seven kids, it only takes a matter of minutes for the house to look this way unless an adult slows up the destruction. If you point out the mess, they look at you as if everything just fell apart as they were passing through the room. I've thought about piping a subliminal message tape throughout the house that would just keep playing the words "Pick it up . . . put it away . . . pick it up . . . put it away."

My heart was pounding hard, and my hands began to get sweaty as I thought about what it was going to actually take mentally and physically for me to pull things together and leave for L.A. that day. I know Linda saw the anxiety on my face, and in her magnificent and intuitive way, she took charge of the moment. She sat me at the kitchen table with the baby and his bottle of formula, and then she turned into a cleaning cyclone. The woman was a blur of motion (or maybe the anxiety was causing my eyes to tremble), scrubbing the countertops, cleaning out the refrigerator, labeling and taping up boxes, shoveling toys and miscellaneous items into their proper places. Everything started to get done, which made me relax, and I gave over control. The best part was, I didn't even have to feel guilty about asking for help. Linda perceived what needed to happen and did it all without even pausing to accept my thanks. She shrugged it off as no big deal, just a little time out of her day. In my eyes, her taking the time to run the vacuum seemed like monumental support, and that act of nurturing helped me see things as manageable. Of all the generous gifts I received that day, hers was the one I needed most.

◆

Late that afternoon, the car was almost at full capacity, with six kids, Netty, who took over as a nanny for Melissa because she was attending a family event, and me behind the wheel. The other car was being driven by Jill, my other great nanny. It was filled to the brim with boxes of things for the L.A. house and had a full U-Haul trailer carrying extra furniture attached behind. My oldest son, Stephen, and his cousin Dominic, had flown to L.A. the day before to be there when the movers arrived at the new house. My business manager, Allen, my personal manager, Karl Engemann, and Lisa had stopped by to have me sign some last-minute papers and say good-bye. The three of them saw the full trailer and the two cars and made a last-attempt plea bargain.

"We know we can't talk you out of driving," Allen said. "But towing a trailer is another matter. It's too dangerous to cross the desert in the summer. What if the car overheats from pulling the extra weight?"

I wasn't thinking "What if?" I was thinking "Why wait?" I tried to calm their apprehensions. I mean, I'd done this drive dozens of times with a car full of kids, and I'd driven everything from a moped to a tour bus. I could handle two cars and a trailer.

Brian called from San Francisco to try to talk me out of driving altogether. He said he would figure it out, and asked me to put my plan on hold until he did. I didn't feel I had the time to waste. There was the house to fix up, and I had to fix myself up as well. I needed to schedule time with my personal trainer to get the extra pounds off before the show started back up. I only had a short time left, so I dismissed Brian's concerns, knowing that I needed to take charge. Just as I was about to pull away in our caravan, he called one more time. "I'm not there to keep you from doing this," he said. "But I'm asking you to leave the packed car and the trailer behind. I'm extremely uncomfortable with you trying to do it this way. Please respect my wishes."

I didn't have the energy to argue about it anymore. He assured me he would find a way to get the trailer to L.A. Jill, who was in the second car, handed over the keys to Allen, squeezed in with the rest of us, and off we went, into the sunset.

As soon as we were on the highway, I found myself feeling more relaxed than I had in weeks. We started to chuckle about how our full car must have looked to others. I started singing the *Beverly Hillbillies* theme, because if Grandma had been along she definitely would have had to sit on top of the car in a rocking chair. Being behind the wheel felt like the first chance I had had in a long time to take a deep breath. It was therapeutic for me, the simplicity of driving, my only purpose being to get to a new destination. I didn't have to do anything else, and I wasn't being pulled in a million different directions. It was great, and the feeling of going eighty-five miles per hour (I mean sixty-five) was totally freeing.

We stopped in Las Vegas for the night. I had called my friend Felix Rappaport, who was then running the MGM Grand hotel. Donny and I have performed at the MGM since we were teenagers, and have always felt at home there. Felix has always gone out of his way to make my family and me feel comfortable, and this time was no exception.

We had a family dinner in the room, and I got the kids settled in their beds for the night. It was so wonderful to have a bit of time to myself that I curled up on the bed to watch a Steve Martin–Goldie Hawn movie, *The Out-of-Towners*. Steve and Goldie play a hapless married couple who go to New York City for a job interview and fall victim to a slew of bad circumstances, from losing their luggage to being mugged to being kicked out of a hotel. I laughed really hard for the first time in what seemed like years. Maybe I was relating too much to feeling out of control and tossed around by circumstances.

I thought I would be exhausted from the baby shower and the long drive, but I actually felt an incredible sense of freedom. I must have wanted the feeling to last, because I stayed up until three A.M. watching movies and laughing.

Early the next morning, I let Jill drive because I knew I probably wasn't as alert as I should have been. The baby had been fussy most of the night and woke the other kids at five in the morning. I decided to take a turn in the car seat row and handed Jill the keys.

From the moment we pulled out of the parking lot I had a strong feeling this wouldn't be an ordinary trip. I tried ignoring it, but it became more intense when we got on the highway. I couldn't stop focusing on the car ahead of us. I repeatedly told Jill to leave more distance between our car and the one in front. I was feeling uneasy about following this car, but I couldn't really say why. Just as I was voicing my concerns again about allowing more braking room, the car ahead of us lost control, screeched across the lane, and flipped over on the median strip, raising a huge cloud of dust and smoke. Another car, one lane over, swerved to miss hitting that car and spun out right in front of us.

We had come within inches of being involved in a massive accident. One of my first thoughts, after giving thanks and making sure everyone was okay, was if we had been towing the trailer, the weight of it probably wouldn't have allowed us to stop in time. Even though we were all safe, I started feeling incredible anxiety again and knew I wouldn't be able to remain calm unless I was the one driving. I drove the rest of the way to Los Angeles, gripping the wheel because I didn't want the kids to see my hands trembling. I tried to tell stories and jokes to keep the atmosphere light, but everyone was shaken. I'd been in close calls before and usually regained my composure quickly. This time the terror of what could have happened stayed with me hour after hour. I tried to focus all my energy on getting us home. I had to take an emotional detour around my battered confidence. I persisted in reassuring everyone that we were safe, but on the inside, my fight-or-flight adrenaline screeched and swerved and flipped my nerves into a crumpled wreck.

11

◆

To See Me This Way

I turned the key in the lock of our new house and pushed the front door open as far as it would go. That was about eight inches. On the other side of the door, blocking the entrance, was our piano. I probably should have taken that as a warning: "Stop now if you want to preserve your last stable nerves. Enter at your own risk." Two of the kids managed to squeeze through the opening and roll the piano far enough away from the door so the rest of us could enter.

What I saw made me want to go right back out and post a garage sale sign in hopes that someone would come along and cart it all away. The couches were wrapped in plastic and stacked one on top of the other. One whole wall of the living room was heaped to the ceiling with boxes and large bags full of clothes and shoes and toys. The mattresses lined another wall, with various headboards, bed frames, and disassembled cribs in between. The kitchen table had miraculously ended up in the right room, but it was stacked with boxes of china, books, and framed photos.

The movers, it seemed, had arrived early, before the freshly cleaned carpets had dried completely. With only my sixteen-year-old there to give directions, they had set everything wherever there were wood floors with empty space. The entrance landing, I guess, had seemed to be the easiest place to ditch the piano.

I stood in the doorway, taking it all in and squelching what could easily have become a full-out scream in my throat. Where did I even start? How was I going to deal with this mess on my own?

I was feeling totally abandoned. This project of unpacking and getting settled was going to be massive, and I couldn't imagine getting through it. I no longer felt patient about Brian's project in San Francisco. I felt he should have been able to perceive how enormous even an everyday task was to me in my weakened emotional and physical state.

I wanted him there with me, though I couldn't seem to let him know that. I repeatedly told him and everyone else who checked in with me that I was fine.

After I walked through the whole house in total shock, trying to make sense of it all, I pulled some boxes down from a stack and started to dig through them, searching for the basics: towels, flatware, drinking glasses.

Earlier in the day, I had talked to my friend Patty Leoni on my cell phone as I was driving into L.A. "I'm glad you're home," Patty told me. "My family is in town and they want to come over to say hello and see the new baby."

She said she could hear in my voice how tired I was and asked if she could help in any way. Again, I even told Patty, my friend since childhood, that I was fine. As comfortable as I was with her family, I was embarrassed by the disarray in my house and I couldn't imagine how I was going to handle having company right away. In true Patty style, she made it as convenient as possible, arriving that evening with buckets of chicken and enough side orders to feed us all. Her mother brought adorable gifts for the baby. We cleared off one end of the kitchen table for the food, located and pulled the plastic wrap off some of the chairs, and gathered to have dinner together, some of us eating picnic style on the floor.

The kids had been very energetic with the excitement of being in a new house, but I could tell they were fading, too. After we finished dinner they started to show signs of being overtired, crying easily and getting on one another's nerves. They needed to go to bed, but the process of arranging the bedrooms was still ahead of us. Patty and I dug through boxes to find sheets, pillows, and quilts, and pulled the mattresses into each of the bedrooms.

By the time Patty left, we had only succeeded in locating and unpacking some plates and glasses, but we couldn't find the flatware or towels for the bathroom. I was too tired to care. I just curled up on my mattress, pulled a comforter over me, and passed out for what seemed like only ten minutes. The toddlers were off their regular schedules and took turns waking me up, wanting to be rocked and held. Once I could get Brandon and Brianna settled, the baby would cry and need to be fed. Every time I went to get back in bed, one of the older kids would have joined the sleepover, telling me they couldn't sleep in their new rooms, and then by the time I had calmed their fears the baby would need to be fed again. At sunrise, we must have looked like a game of Twister gone awry, with seven people on one bed and limbs protruding every which way. I think Stephen was the only one who had a decent night's sleep, because he stayed in his room downstairs.

The next morning Stephen took charge and enlisted the over-age-eight crowd in helping him set up the kitchen. It was a sweet gesture, but let me tell you, finding your way through a kitchen arranged by kids can be an endless and frustrating task. It's like when you try to leave the house quickly and you have your car keys but can't find your wallet. Then you find the wallet and now you've lost the car keys. That was my kitchen. Okay, I've found one saucepan, where could the matching lid be? Under the kitchen sink with the cleanser and scouring pads, of course. The spice jars were parked inside the hot chocolate mugs, and the steak knives were in between the cookie sheets. I have to say it did get the first laugh out of me since our arrival.

I continued sorting through the mounds of boxes and bags in the living room. I think I became obsessed with getting the house in order because everything else in my life felt so chaotic. By the late afternoon, my body started sending up surrender flags: My head was pounding, and my shoulder and neck were beginning to hurt again. Everything I looked at and touched seemed to be shaking up and down rapidly, as if I were hanging on to a jackhammer. I could also tell that my body had not been given time to fully heal from the birth, and I'm sure I wasn't helping myself in the least by lifting and carrying boxes. The noise of the kids talking loudly or the baby crying felt like a siren going off next to my head.

Opening a box and deciding where the contents belonged seemed to be a more staggering task than learning *The King and I* in seventeen days. It felt almost impossible to keep up, with the kids asking me as each box was opened: "Mom, where does this go?" "Who gets this desk lamp?" "Where's my *Star Wars* collection?" "My tap shoes?" "The blanket Grandma made me?"

The phone had been ringing constantly since nine that morning. Every message was a request for time in my schedule, from school enrollments, dance classes, and piano lessons to doll signings, magazine interviews, and meetings for the second season of *Donny & Marie*.

When it was time to feed the baby, I would shut myself

in the bathroom for twenty minutes to be able to spend time with him and to rest for a while myself. While I fed him I would sit on the floor and cry until some of the pressure in my head was released. Then I would try to appear normal again and go back out into the confusion. I didn't want the kids to see me upset, but I think they could tell anyway. My usual way to take on a big job is to jump in feet first and attack with an attitude of "We have to do this, so let's make it fun." But I wasn't that way at all. I was starting to be very short-tempered and impatient with them. The kids were having whispered conversations away from me and giving each other the "watch out" looks that I usually saw thirty minutes after the pizza boxes had been carried out to the trash.

If I eat too much wheat, I usually have an allergic reaction. I can eat it every now and then, but an overload, like pizza, will result in my feeling frazzled and ill for about an hour. The reaction usually makes me irritable. The kids know when this happens and call it a "wheaty." They signal one another to stay away from Mom for an hour because she's having a wheaty. It seemed Mom had been on an endless wheaty since coming home from the hospital.

I had packed large plastic containers with baby blankets and clothes from Utah, and I asked two of the older kids to carry them up the stairs and into the nursery room. When I looked up, I saw that they had piled the containers along the banister on the second level. In my mind all I could see was how easy it would be for one of the toddlers to climb up on the stack and fall over the banister. My reaction to this was severe. What should have been a reprimand for a careless action turned into an emotional torrent that left the kids speechless.

I couldn't believe it was me being like that. I am adamantly against shouting or speaking harshly to another person. I don't like it when my children speak negatively to or belittle one another, even when they claim to be just teasing. I personally think it causes an injury to the soul that is long lasting. Even when the initial pain is gone, the scar of insecurity remains in the memory.

That night at dinner, I sat at the table unable to eat or even talk, which I'm sure made the kids feel uneasy. They filled the silence with kid-type "Yes, it is," "No, it isn't" banter. The chatter escalated into larger arguments and whining. Finally, I called for an end to it. Stephen was the next person to speak, and whatever he said, as harmless as it probably was, turned out to be all I could take. I stood up and slammed my plate to the table (not much of an effect with paper). I remember letting him have it, yelling for what seemed like a full minute. Then I went upstairs to my bedroom and shut the door. I was instantly overcome by great guilt, followed by tears. Stephen had been present all day, helping me organize and overseeing the other children. He has always been a source of strength for me, even from his birth. So I was just as shocked by my explosion as I'm sure he was. In all of my sixteen years with Stephen, I had never had a reason to raise my voice at him to that extreme, and whatever he had said at the dinner table certainly did not deserve that response.

The baby was sleeping in the bassinet next to my bed. Looking at his tiny face gave me huge feelings of regret. I started questioning myself: "What is wrong with you? What are you becoming? Why can't you get through this? Your children depend on you. You have to be strong for them. So many women are less blessed than you are and they don't fall apart!"

Waves of anger crashed over me. I punished myself with repeated messages of worthlessness. I was talking to myself in the exact way I would not allow my children to speak to one another. The fearful inner me needed to be taken care of and nurtured, but the outer me pushed, bullied, and taunted my weak inner self. It was like trying to march out of quicksand; I was only going deeper in. My heart was already engulfed in heaviness, and I could feel the darkness swallowing any logic I had left and choking off the will to struggle to firm ground.

Again, I reached for the only lifeline I could think of. I called Brian in San Francisco. I had to let him know I was battling desperation and losing. The feeling of despondency is lonely, and a difficult one to share, even with those who love you. It takes over your whole being. You exist in a world that is business as usual: restaurants are full, companies are operating, people are shopping, working, studying, and some are producing CDs. While all of life is going on, you feel isolated, pushed out. It's hard to ask for help, and harder yet to have others comprehend where you are.

When Brian answered the phone, I told him what was going on with the house and I said, "I really can't take all of this right now."

He responded, "I knew I shouldn't have taken this project. I was planning to do some music editing in Utah, but if you really need me, I'll come home."

I couldn't even believe what came out of my mouth next. "No," I responded, going numb by the second. "No. I'm fine. Fine."

I couldn't even say yes to my husband's offer of help. I was betraying myself and for the first time I could see it. I didn't want him to ask if I needed him. I wanted him to know I needed him. I was too hurt to say yes, so I swallowed it, betraying my true feelings. I swallowed it because I wanted him to decide on his own to come home. Feeling as I did about this, there wasn't a chance I was going to say that I needed help. I would handle it on my own. I'd figure it out. I had always managed before and I would somehow do it again.

I hung up the phone and tried to bring myself back to reality. I felt a deep chill come over me, as if my life were draining away. I went to get a sweater from my closet. The closet looked dark and hidden, and without thought I crawled in and sat on the floor in the corner. It was where I would retreat as a child when I felt hurt, frightened, or confused. Now here I was again. I began to cry hard, muffling the noise of my sobs with clothes hanging nearby. Then, suddenly, the out-of-control crying stopped and I sat silently in the darkness, with just tears running from my eyes. I lost a total sense of myself and complete track of time. I heard my daughter calling, "Mom?" into the room, but I couldn't respond. I could feel myself crossing the fine line that separates reality from illusion. I was letting go of myself, and I didn't care. I don't think I moved again until the baby woke up, and his cries of hunger were the only thing that put the brakes on my descent. I know that his true helplessness without me was the only thing that kept me attached to reality. I was brought back from the edge and somehow forced to function again. Almost as if my body stood apart from my mind, I got up, put on a sweater, gathered up my baby, and headed downstairs to fix his bottle.

The kids had cleared the table and were cautiously checking out my mood as I came down the stairs. I wanted to take them in my arms and reassure them, but real life had resumed again. In my living room stood my new next-door neighbor. She had brought over a plate of baked goods to welcome us to the neighborhood. I remember her saying, "Let me know if there's anything you need."

I'm sure I probably smiled automatically, but my response was "All I really want is to be left alone."

I could hear the words coming out of my mouth, so I knew it was me talking, but I couldn't believe I was really saying that to a woman I didn't even know and who was extending herself to make me feel welcome. I would never talk like that to someone who didn't know me. But my mouth had taken over and was committed to the words. Even my daughter Rachael was looking at me as if to ask, "Who are you? What did you do with my mother?"

Even though I cared that I had most likely offended my new neighbor and even hurt her feelings, I had nothing left in me to do damage control. Since then, I have apologized to this woman, who later told me, "I had no idea how much pain you were in. You looked so in control." That day, I think she handed the plate of goodies to my daughter and made a quick retreat out the front door.

The two nannies, Jill and Netty, who had made the trip from Utah to L.A. with us, worked hard helping me organize the kids so I could get the house settled. After I fed the baby, Jill, not knowing of my currently fragmented emotional state, picked that time to tell me she needed a day off to take care of personal things.

I remember looking at her face as if she were requesting the impossible, and I don't think I even answered her. I went back upstairs to my bedroom because I could feel myself completely falling apart inside. I laid the baby down and knelt at the edge of the bed. I wasn't sure I had spirit left in me to pray, but I couldn't think of doing anything else. As I knelt there, I kept thinking of how I had lost my sense of humor, refused help from my husband, yelled at my kids, and collapsed, hidden away from everyone, in my closet. I thought about my reaction to Jill's request for time off and how I had told my neighbor that I just wanted to be alone. I realized, at that moment, that I had actually been speaking the truth. I should be alone. I was not a person who should be around children because I couldn't stop crying, I was impatient, in pain, angry, and unable to control what I was saying. I was a mess. I thought, "No one deserves to be around me like this: not the neighbor, not the baby-sitters, and especially not my children." It was then that I knew I had to leave until I could come to terms with what was happening to me. I couldn't let my children continue to see me this way.

I picked myself up off the floor, found my purse, and took out my wallet. I tore out three blank checks and signed them. I then took out a credit card and my bank card. I threw the wallet back in my bag and gathered the baby from the bed.

I walked down the stairs and put my precious baby in Netty's arms. I put the checks and the cards in her hand and said, "Please understand that I couldn't do this if I didn't have you here. I can't stay. There is something wrong, really wrong with me, and I have to leave until I figure it out. Brian is at this number. Call him. He'll come home."

Netty looked at me with a stunned expression and asked if I was okay.

"No," I said, without holding back. "No. I'm not."

I turned away from her, away from my baby, and away from my life, and walked out the door.

I have no idea how my feet carried me to the car. I turned the key in the ignition, put the car in reverse, and backed down the driveway. When I shifted into drive, something overpowering moved inside of me, from the deepest part of my soul. My body was racked with hysterical crying and I began to understand for the first time why a person would want to take their own life.

12

$\Diamond$

A Final Plea

The beauty of the California coast was created by violent shifts of the earth a long time ago. The rolling foothills that are now covered with orchards or wildflowers stand where steaming lava once spilled into the ocean. Jagged cliffs hang overhead on the right as you drive north along the coast. On the left, ocean waves pound down on the sandy bluffs. It can be both spectacular and frightening. At nature's whim, a chunk of mountain could topple down onto the four-lane highway, or a storm-sized wave could crash over the guardrail. Everything in your surroundings is both bigger and more powerful than you are. Logically, it doesn't make sense that a road was ever built through this area, let alone lasted to this day. Considering the odds of a mishap it was probably wrong to clear access for cars along the rugged coast, but when you're driving on it, taking in the view, it feels right.

Twenty minutes after backing out of my driveway, I was on the Pacific Coast Highway, heading north. I wasn't taking in the view. I probably couldn't have told anyone where I was. I wasn't focused on direction. I was thinking, "I've left my home and my children and I'm driving away from everything: the pressure, the pain, and the responsibility. I want relief from my life. And though I am sure this is wrong, it feels right. It feels right that I should be alone, because I can't think of a single person to call. Whom could I trust to understand? I don't even understand. Who would want to be with me the way I am? I've become a miserable person who should be left alone. It feels right that I am leaving, because my children deserve to have a mother who is truly there for them, one who is emotionally stable, strong, and happy. It feels right that as I drive the sky is changing from dusk into dark, because I am dark. There is no light, no joy anywhere in me. I'm completely alone.

I somehow maneuvered the turns in the road, which seemed more threatening in the dark but not nearly as threatening as my thoughts. I contemplated that life might be easier for everyone I loved if I were not on this earth. In the past, I had never understood why a person would make the choice to end his or her life. I always saw it as such a waste because I believe we each have a purpose. I can now comprehend how much a lack of self-worth affects that decision. If you don't see yourself as counting for anything, then you also don't see it as a waste if you were to no longer exist.

I believe that God never gives us more than we can handle. I was feeling at the very outer edge of what I could manage, but I never doubted that God was with me. I believe that he gave me life and that when it should end is ultimately his decision, but I still found it difficult to understand why there was purpose in existing as I was. I felt useless.

My tears poured out continuously as I drove.

I have heard people who have gone through near-death experiences describe how their lives played out before them in what seemed to be their final moments. I could tell that my heart continued to beat, my eyes could see, and my hands could still steer the car, but a form of death was taking place. There was an abandoned and injured child buried alive deep inside of me, and this was her final cry for help. I was experiencing the type of hysteria you might find in a lost little girl, one who has been separated from the security of anything familiar to her. I felt like a child who had tried to fit in, to be acknowledged, but who had been told her whole life, "Not now. I don't have time for you." Now she was there to beg for my attention, and I could no longer ignore the feelings. I let myself open up to how frightened this little girl was and how lost she had been feeling for so many years.

I had not allowed myself to experience many of my true emotions since I was small. They had become deep secrets that I kept, even from myself. After all, emotions are too unpredictable and sloppy to be allowed to exist in the life of a One-Take Osmond.

Mile after mile, as I was driving up the coast, long-forgotten experiences came back to my memory. Ages three, five, seven, nine, thirteen: feelings of being scared, overwhelmed, demoralized, and abused. I thought about the long months of being on the road with so many different people, and my family being the only consistency and safe connection in my life. I pictured the controlling adults, those with short-term investments in our careers, surrounding me with critical and oppressive attention. I could sense, as if it were happening again right then, the frightening and manipulative abuse by those who were supposed to have had my best interests in mind. I wept in anguish as these dark thoughts crept up from the tomb of my memory.

Ages fourteen, sixteen, nineteen, twenty: being scrutinized, criticized, and sexualized. My thoughts took me to the negative gossip and feedback I read or heard about my family, my recording career, and the television show. I remembered hearing the snide remarks of those who found fault with my career moves. Every time such a knife was thrown, I had been encouraged to shrug it off or take it in stride. But knives can't be shrugged off, and each one had left a deeper wound, infecting me with self-anger and the feeling that I would never be good enough. I grieved about all the money from the first *Donny & Marie* show that had been lost through poor advice, much of it during the years that my parents had entrusted our finances to others while they were serving a mission for our church. I remembered the anxious feeling of having to sell everything we owned and start over again to spare our family the necessity of declaring bankruptcy.

I felt gut-wrenching anger about having nothing to show for four years of working eighty-hour weeks during my lost childhood. I had taxed myself to the limit to be what I thought the entertainment industry wanted, and for what? I thought about the subtle but constant pressure to be mature beyond my years, and then, after the original *Donny & Marie* show had been cancelled, feeling tossed aside because I was no longer a hot commodity. I felt dismissed and then ignored as a has-been at age twenty.

Ages twenty-four, twenty-six, thirty-one, thirty-five, thirty-eight: a failed marriage, being a single mom and having to care and provide for my son, taking care of my employees, taking home the paycheck, proving to the country music industry that I could deliver another string of hit songs, going on the road with such a full schedule of shows that my immune system eventually collapsed. What started as a bad case of mono had side effects that stayed with me for almost four years. I remembered the stress of having to scramble to reinvent myself, from country music to a sitcom, from Broadway productions to the talk show, and many projects in between. I let myself mourn over the instability caused by relocating so many times, from Utah to Nashville, from New York to Los Angeles, and the effect it had on my children. I felt deep sorrow about the long-term effects that years of radical dieting in order to look right had had on my body. Even on the new *Donny & Marie* show, I felt the same pressure about my appearance. I resented the rumor mill that picked me apart as a person, from my marriage to being a mother.

I had thought I was beyond those hurts, that I had willed them away, focusing on my work and burying them deep inside of me so they'd never surface. I had been convinced that I had become stronger by labeling them as petty feelings and casting them out of my consciousness. I had thought they had been safely put six feet under and could "rest in peace." I had moved forward, making the best of it all. I was so unaware of the cumulative effect of all my buried emotions.

For thirty-seven years I had denied this inner self, the little girl I had submerged in the name of practicality so long ago. Now, driving up the coast, she was shouting it all out and making it clear that she was suffocating and there was no chance of survival unless I paid attention right now. No more hiding. No more denial. No more pain.

◆

Something else was demanding my attention too . . . a cell phone. As I drove, I could hear it somewhere in the car, ringing persistently.

Stephen had borrowed my car to go out on a date the night before. I had asked him to take my cell phone in case something happened or I needed to get ahold of him. He had tucked it behind the front passenger sun visor and forgotten to bring it back in the house. When I gave it to him, I couldn't have predicted that twenty-four hours later he would be wondering if something had happened to me, and be worried enough to call Brian in San Francisco. Brian got that call while he was at the airport waiting to board a flight to Utah. After Stephen told him of my sudden departure, he caught the next flight into L.A. instead.

I'm not sure how long I was aware of the phone ringing. I don't think I could identify what it was for quite some time; it just seemed like some type of background noise. Finally, frustrated by the constant ringing, I found it and answered. Brian was on the other end. He sounded relieved to hear my voice, but I was not ready to hear his.

I told him I didn't know where I was going and I hung up. The phone began to ring again immediately. I answered it. Brian was trying to figure out where I was by engaging me in conversation. I couldn't speak because I was crying so hard, and I could barely listen. I had shut down; I had too much going on in my own head to hear his thoughts about what I was doing. I hung up the phone. It rang again right away, and the cycle would repeat: Brian would attempt to pinpoint my location, asking me about nearby landmarks and highway signs, and try to reason with me. Trying to understand what he was saying or answer his questions left me feeling confused and mentally exhausted. I would tell him that I could only see darkness and that I wanted to be left alone. I would hang up and let the phone ring without answering it. I could have turned it off completely, and was tempted to throw it out the window at fifty-five miles an hour, as Brianna had done, but I didn't out of fear, because I knew somewhere inside of me that this phone was my last link to my sanity.

The vastness of the dark ocean beside me seemed so peaceful compared to what I was feeling. I pulled off at the next exit and drove down to the beach. When Brian called again, I told him I was going for a walk. He was very agitated and vocal about this choice. Over and over again he said, "Stay in the car, Marie. You have to be smart. Lock the doors. It's very late and too dangerous to walk on the beach."

I stayed in the car and on the phone, listening to his voice but not responding much at all. I knew walking by myself in the middle of the night was unwise, but I didn't want to be told what to do anymore. I became angrier by the minute. I had listened and followed instructions and directions my whole life. Where had that led me? Was I even my own person, or just a composite of what others had created me to be?

I don't know how much time passed while I sat in the car, staring out at the ocean, listening to Brian's voice on the phone but not responding. Because I agreed to stay in the car, my anger only increased. I was still following instructions, doing what I was told. For my entire life, I thought, I've placed my opinion below that of other people.

I started up the car and got back on the highway. I think Brian hoped I would head back to Los Angeles, but I continued north, making my way along the coast of California. I didn't know specifically where I was. I didn't care, either. I only cared that it was my choice to keep going.

The next time Brian called, he pleaded with me, "Please, if you don't want to come back, at least pull off and stay in a hotel for the night. You shouldn't be driving when you're this upset."

I didn't want to stop, because I felt if I couldn't be in control of my life, I could at least be in control of the car. I had no plans to return home until I had figured out what was wrong with me.

Some time later, I was listening to Brian on the phone when the road narrowed and suddenly I was fast approaching a cement divider that seemed to come from nowhere. It was being used to separate the road for a construction project, but I never saw the warning signs. I dropped the phone on the floor, screamed, and grabbed the wheel, narrowly missing a head-on collision with the pillar. Brian was terrified, thinking I had been in an accident but not knowing for sure because the call had disconnected when the phone fell. There was no place for me to pull over because the shoulder of the road was blocked off with dividers. I could hear the phone ringing again, but I was shaking and too afraid to take my hands off the wheel for even a few seconds to reach down to find it on the floor.

When I finally regained enough composure to locate the phone and answer it, Brian was both relieved and even more adamant about my stopping and finding a hotel room for the night. By this time I was bleary eyed and my arms ached from the tension of grasping the wheel for so long. I agreed to pull off the highway at the next safe exit and find a place. I still had no idea where I was or that I had traveled almost 250 miles from L.A.

I came upon a small roadside motel, more of a truckers' stopover. I didn't look to see what the name of it was or even what town I was in. I have no memory of even going to the front desk. I was given a room on the ground floor, which had a parking lot entrance and a sliding door opening onto a dark courtyard. I remember thinking that it was probably not a safe place to be alone, but I didn't care. Brian had told me to call him as soon as I was in a room.

When he answered the phone he started questioning me: "Where are you? What's the name of the hotel?"

I said, "I have no idea."

"Then look at the phone," he pleaded, "and give me the number."

"Please," I said. "Listen to me. I'm not coming back."

"Don't hang up. Look for the phone number so I can figure out where you are."

My eyes were so tired that I could not focus them enough to see a number on the phone, but he kept insisting that I look one more time. Finally, I found the phone number and read it to him.

"I'll come to get you," Brian told me.

"No. I'm fine," I responded.

Again I betrayed my true feelings, and again Brian took me literally. "Go to sleep now and I'll come for you in the morning," he said.

At that moment, I didn't really care if he came to get me or not. I knew I hadn't told him what I really needed, but I was deeply hurt that he couldn't see through what I was saying and insist that he was coming right now anyway. I didn't believe there was any way he would be able to help me deal with my situation or truly comprehend how serious it was.

I lay down on the bed and tried to sleep, but my thoughts were agonizingly harsh. "Why would I be given my life if I couldn't handle it? What kind of mother am I? How could I be so selfish? Here I had seven beautiful children, a thirteen-year marriage, and a long-lasting career, so many things that other people would love to have. My mother raised nine kids and coped with a life on the road. She didn't fall apart. Why am I such a failure? Why am I in so much pain? What will happen to my babies? What have I done? Why am I so weak? My hardships are nothing like ones that other people handle: illness, disability, lack of family support, and severe financial struggles. And where am I? In a dark motel room hundreds of miles from my family."

My self-hatred grew by the minute. I didn't feel worthy of what I had. I wasn't thankful for my great life. I felt as if there wasn't one redeemable quality in who I was.

I dropped to my knees at the edge of the bed for the only prayer I could manage. "Help me," I pleaded. "I can't find any way out of this darkness. I'm so weary. I can't do it."

I curled up in a ball on the bed and I slept. I couldn't tell if it was for fifteen minutes or for an hour or two, but when I woke up it was still dark outside. My heart was pounding, and I was completely confused. Once I figured out where I was, I wanted to get back in my car and drive again. I was so listless, and my insides felt as though they were on fire. My neck was in spasm with sharp, shooting pain similar to the way it had felt in the emergency room. I couldn't fall back to sleep. I remembered that I still had some prescription pain pills left from my trip to the hospital and that they were probably still in my purse. I went out to the car and found my purse, which I had left on the backseat. I sat with the bottle in my hand thinking how easy it would be for me to take them all and be done with it. But with my belief system that would never be an option. More than that, I thought about not being there to put my arms around my children if they were in pain and needed comforting. What deep wounds and sorrows would be left for them to deal with because I wanted to end my pain.

I remember saying out loud to myself, "Marie. You're pathetic." I thought about driving again, just to try to escape my self-pity. Instead, I took two of the pills even though the label said one, locked the car, and went back into the room. I was thinking, "Just sleep. Sleep and you won't have to feel for a while."

It was daylight when Brian had a friend drop him off at the motel. I could hear him knocking on the door for a while, but I didn't want to let him in the room. Finally I answered the door, but I still couldn't respond much when he talked to me. I felt I was far back behind my eyes, hiding and floating. It was like looking at him through a heat wave. Everything was distorted. There was no way that he could reach me. I think he tried to talk to me most of the morning, and then at one point he took me in his arms and just held on to me and started to cry. That was the first moment I felt even an ounce of life come back into my body, but I had no tears left to shed.

He said, "I love you. I'm here for you. I'm not going anywhere. I will see you through this."

I knew he meant it sincerely, but I still couldn't find a way to respond. Even when he curled up next to me on the bed, I turned my back to him. I didn't want him near.

At some point, Brian called my parents. I could hear him talking to my father, but I couldn't comprehend what was being said. I just lay on the bed, staring at the wall, feeling as if I were not really in the room but in a far-off place from which I would never return. Then Brian put the phone to my ear, and my father said, "I love you. Your mother wants to talk to you." I next heard my mother say my name. The sound of her voice did something to me, brought my attention back into the moment. It was my mom. The little girl in me started to listen and respond.

But my mother wasn't waiting for me to respond. She was rescuing her baby, reaching through the pain to soothe and comfort me as only she can.

I could hear the sadness and worry in her voice.

"Marie, you'll be okay," she said reassuringly. "I know what you're going through, sweetheart. I really do. Listen, I'm going to tell you something I've never told anyone about me."

I felt myself connect with her as if she were there with me, right next to my bed, stroking my hair.

"I was almost your age when I had my last baby," she said. "Not only had I just given birth, but we had also picked up and moved the whole family to California. Your father had given up his job in Utah because the kids were starting their weekly appearances on *The Andy Williams Show*. We had moved into a new house. Everything was different about our lives, and I was worried about all the risks involved with show business and the long-term effect it would have on all of you. I remember saying, 'This is too much. I feel completely overworked and underappreciated.' I handed the baby to your father and told him, 'I have to get out of here.' Then I got in the car and I drove up the coast."

I remember opening my eyes and sitting halfway up on the bed. Did she say "drove up the coast"?

I could barely say anything to her because I was choked with emotion. For the first time since the baby was born I felt a true release. I put my head back down on the pillow with the phone pressed to my ear and whispered to her, "Mommy, I'm so sad."

"It will get better," my mother consoled me. "You'll be all right again. Trust me. I know you will."

My hope started to grow just a bit because I did trust her, so I knew I wasn't losing my mind. She had once felt this way and I knew she wasn't crazy. If she had overcome it, then perhaps I could too.

That conversation marked a turning point in my worst moments of postpartum depression. My mother made me feel I could go on. She had no instant cure to offer or great advice that made the light break through for me. She merely had an admission. She simply said that she knew what I was going through. There was someone who really understood, and it was my mother. It changed my path.

I began to feel relieved and I think I even smiled when she said, "Like mother, like daughter."

I said, "I love you," and handed the phone to Brian.

After that phone call, I rested for a couple of hours.

I could tell Brian was exhausted from being afraid for so long. He had never seen me like this before, but he wasn't alone. I had never seen me like this either.

Finally, as evening approached, Brian said, "You can't

stay in this room forever. You really will rest better at home. We have to go back, Marie, so the kids will know you're all right. They need you."

Those words hit me hard. My children needed me. A substitute would not work. I could almost hear them saying to me, "Mommy, I'm so sad," in the way I had said it to my own mother. She had been there for me. Now I should be there for my own children.

I still wanted to stay hidden away, but I decided that the only thing to do was go home. I would take care of my babies and try to exist as best I could. So once again I shut down my own feelings. I stood up to leave with Brian. Before he pulled the door closed on the motel room, I turned around to look at it, the scrubby little refuge where I had learned to listen to my own heart for a few hours. Then, through my whole being, I sensed a final plea from the banished little girl inside of me, whom I was pushing away again: "You still didn't take care of me!"

13

---◆---

One Shoe In

I was home. I had been found and returned. I was with my husband and my children. That was where I was needed, where I should be. I was there, but I was completely absent. I don't remember what time it was when Brian and I got back home. I don't remember anything about the two or three days that followed. I don't remember what I was feeling.

Memory is connected with feeling. I think we remember events and moments because of the feelings we connect with them. I had shut my feelings down so completely that I was just surviving in time and space.

I had no expectations. I didn't expect my life to return to normal. I didn't expect my children to want to be around me ever again. I didn't expect my husband to know how or what to do to help me and I couldn't even let him try. I didn't expect anyone to understand the reason I had left.

My only hopeful thought was: "My mother went through this. Maybe I can get through too."

I gripped this thought and replayed it in my mind over and over. I've always thought of my mother as a much stronger person than I am, so I wasn't completely convinced that my experience would resolve the way hers had. But I clung to the possibility. I was like a drowning woman, hanging on to that one thin string to keep from going under completely.

◆

Iknow how much my mother influenced my whole life. Over the years, whenever everything else in my life was in motion, I could count on her presence to be steady. When she went through a rough time, was not feeling well, or was upset, I could pick up on it even though she didn't want anyone to know. Even now, there is little that unsettles me more than knowing something is not all right with my mother. She and I spoke after my return from the coast about the effect her driving off may have had on me at age three. Knowing my deep connection with her, it's hard to believe that I would have remained untouched by her emotional state, even at such a young age.

I try to be conscious of what my children pick up from me. I weigh the influence everything I say and do has on my children. All the major decisions I've made in my adult life, from business choices to personal ones, have been guided by my love for my kids. They're why I got in the car to drive up the coast. I felt it was better that I be absent than to have my babies suffer any instability and insecurity because of my absent state of mind. I think you can convince the public, your friends, and even extended family members that you're getting by fine, but it's impossible to fool your children for very long. Little ones have a great instinct for recognizing insincerity and will point it out before you can finish saying the words "Everything's fine." I could only imagine how I would have felt as a little girl, seeing my mother fall apart emotionally before my eyes. She, like many women, was the one who picked up the pieces of everything else that broke. She's the root from which I felt grounded and secure enough to grow and branch out. The choices she made while raising me are the mainstay of how I mother my own children and the basis by which I approach all of life.

◆

My doll business grew from a hobby my mother started me on when I was a small girl. Together we collected dolls from wherever we toured around the world. I was her only daughter, so dolls and the color pink were very present in my life. As an adult, I've let go of most of the pink but kept the dolls. Now she has enough granddaughters to overdose with pink.

When I make an appearance on television retailer QVC or in a store that carries my line of dolls, I have the pleasure of seeing the bridge a doll can provide between people. I've had mothers tell me that collecting gives them a common bond with their preteen daughters. I've had fathers bring their daughters to a doll signing, grandmothers pick out dolls for their grandchildren, sisters who collect together, and husbands who shop for their wives. I've received letters from collectors who met each other at a doll signing and have ended up becoming close friends.

But I was having a hard time feeling happy about my upcoming appearance on QVC, which was scheduled to take place six days after my journey up the coast. I didn't really want to think about dolls. I still felt my emotions were unpredictable, and my body continued to retain large amounts of fluid from my pregnancy. Every day I had tried to convince myself that I could tough it out and get ready to go back to work. Every night I found that it was all I could do to drag myself around the house and help figure out some sort of meal for everyone. It was usually some kind of easy-to-fix food that I knew everyone liked: macaroni and cheese, soup, pizza, or, many more nights than I'd like to admit, fast food from a drive through. I didn't have any of the focus it took to plan meals ahead of time.

Two days before I was to fly to Philadelphia for the QVC appearance, I was forced to face the fact that I was not back in shape enough to fit into anything I had that was appropriate to wear on television. I was going to have to do some last-minute shopping. I couldn't even imagine walking into a department store, to say nothing of trying on clothing. But I had no choice.

I left my house with great apprehension, headed for one of my favorite department stores. My longtime musical director and composer, Jerry Williams, and his wife, Wendy, have been friends of ours for many years. Wendy is a buyer for that store. I wasn't aware of it, but Brian had called ahead and asked Wendy if she had any time to help me. Did I ever need help! Wendy found me on the first floor, staring at a makeup counter, completely baffled by what I needed to accomplish. Can you believe it? Me, the queen of makeup advice for others, had no idea what to buy. It was so comforting to have Wendy take charge for me, like being lost while driving around a big city in a foreign country and then having a friend appear who says, "Follow me. I'll show you the way."

Wendy took me gently by the arm and said, "We'll get you all set up. Let's start with panty hose." For over two hours, she took me around the store, helping me select clothes to try on, even having an alteration person do a quick fitting on the jackets we selected. She arranged for them to be ready for me to pick up on my way to the airport. I couldn't seem to thank her enough. What probably would have reduced me to tears in minutes, Wendy turned into a productive and calming experience. Brian knew I would need some assistance, but Wendy went beyond that request. She really took care of me.

The next morning, I was sitting in a terminal at the Los Angeles airport as they were making final boarding calls for my flight to Philadelphia, where QVC broadcasts are taped. I couldn't move. I sat near the gate, the baby in my arms, but I couldn't make myself get on the plane. I was weighed down by more than my figure; I was heavy with worry and panic. It was only four weeks after the birth of my baby and less than a week since my drive up the coast. It was also less than twenty-four hours since I stood at a makeup counter, unable to remember what I needed or even how to ask for help. All of this, coupled with my concern about flying with the baby for the first time, left me drenched in fear that I wouldn't be able to cope. A weekend full of QVC shows, as enjoyable as they are, always takes every ounce of energy, even when I'm feeling great.

But I had made a commitment to QVC and I had to appear. It was a "Today's Special Value" appearance, which meant I would go on the air periodically throughout a twenty-four-hour day to show the featured doll. All shows on QVC are planned a year in advance so the dolls can be produced and shipped to QVC on time. They handle such a high quantity of products that reshuffling the schedule is impossible.

The income of other people—sculptors, salespeople, order takers, on-air hosts, and even the people who constructed the dolls and their accessories—depended on my showing up. I cared about these people, so it was never a question of whether I would go, it was a question of whether I could pull it off once I got there.

Usually I fly to all of my appearances with my longtime manager, Karl Engemann. I'm sure if he had been with me at the airport, he would have known exactly what to say to allay my fears and help me get on the plane. Sometimes Karl understands me better than I do. He has been my personal manager for twenty-eight years and has guided me through almost every career change in my life since my adolescence. He had proven to be a man of honor, a person I have completely trusted and also leaned on. If you've spotted me in the audience at award shows and noticed a striking man with a mane of snow white hair sitting next to me, that's Karl.

Maureen FitzPatrick, the co-executive producer of *Donny & Marie*, nicknamed Karl "the Godfather" because of his handsome Marlon Brando looks and the way he always takes care of and protects his family. That family includes Brian and me and all of our children, as well as our office staff and the other people who work closely with me. The trials and joys Karl and I have gone through together could fill a book of their own. We've had both exhilarating and humorous times together. The crazy things that have happened can still make me laugh, from his bout of diet-soda amnesia to a painful charley horse at a formal awards banquet followed by a dignified exit with two plates of dessert. I would tell you the full stories, but he has too many on me that he could bring up as payback. I think, in part, we've survived together for so many years because of his excellent sense of humor. And because he knows that I'm always right . . . did I say sense of humor? I've always known how blessed I am to have such an astute businessman, loyal guide, and friend in my life through my whole career.

But this time I was traveling on my own. Both Lisa Hatch and Karl had flown out of Salt Lake City and planned to meet me in Philadelphia. I could see the ticket taker at the airline desk motioning to me that the door would be closing momentarily and that my time to board was running out. Total panic set in.

I wanted to close my eyes, then open them to find that I was sleeping and the nightmare was over. But that was an empty wish, so I faced the moment ahead by thinking, "Right now I need to get on the airplane." Somehow, I remembered the scene in the movie *What About Bob?* in which Bill Murray stands up and moves forward by saying out loud to himself, "Baby step. Baby step. Baby step." I took my mind off my fears long enough for me to put one foot forward, then the other, until I made it to my seat.

Lisa had told me that she had arranged for a car and a driver to meet me at the gate so I would have help with the baby and my luggage. As chance would have it, the driver met Lisa at her gate in a different terminal. I knew that was probably what had happened when he didn't appear, so I set up the stroller for the baby, who was fussy and hungry, and went to baggage claim and got a luggage cart. I found my bags and loaded them, then I pushed the cart and the baby's stroller to the terminal where Lisa's flight was coming in.

As many times as I've flown, I would normally just take something like this, a glitch in the plans, in stride. This time, it seemed like a huge ordeal that frazzled my nerves completely. Keeping an eye on the baby, pushing the stroller and the luggage cart, and figuring out where to find Lisa seemed insurmountable. By the time I found her and got into the car, I was spent and weepy, and I still had to face the working hours that were ahead of me.

Lisa and I were both hoping we would be able to relax for a couple of hours once we got to the hotel, until I went to hang up my clothes. I had obviously had a hard time packing that morning. I guess trying to put together everything I would need and what I had to pack for the baby had consumed the few brain cells that were still functioning. I had forgotten to pack panty hose and hair spray, and even worse,

I had only packed one shoe! And I had to be ready to attend a doll collectors' dinner in less than two hours.

I knocked on Lisa's door and said, "You'll never believe what I forgot!"

Lisa, who's always fast with a comeback, stood in the doorway and said, "Marie, did you leave the baby at the airport?"

"No, I left my brain in the delivery room," I said, holding up the one shoe as proof. "Do you think they could FedEx the other one to me in two hours?"

Some emergency shopping was called for again. I think I just pointed to a pair of shoes, said, "In a seven" and "Visa," and went back to the hotel.

◆

The next morning, I was not in a good frame of mind from the moment I got up. I had done an on-air appearance from midnight to one A.M. the night before and had to be back at the studio at six-thirty A.M. to arrange the order of the dolls we were going to debut and write out my notes for each doll. My hairstylist, Connie, was eager and happy to watch Matthew for me. I was due back on the air at nine A.M., with other appearances scheduled almost hourly throughout the day. Everything that was a part of my normal routine became a struggle. The makeup I had bought the day before couldn't hide how tired I was. Lisa and I would go over our notes together and then five minutes later I couldn't remember any of it. It was so unlike me that I was overcome by feelings of inadequacy and anxiety about going on the air.

About fifteen minutes before my appearance, Lisa and I were in the dressing room reviewing the information again, when my hands started to tremble uncontrollably. I was short of breath and broke into a cold sweat. My legs wouldn't hold me up, and I collapsed to the floor.

Lisa tried to help me up, telling me I was just a little nervous, but I said to her, "I can't do this. I can't go on."

"Yes, you can, Marie. You can do QVC in your sleep," Lisa said in an attempt to ease my panic. "You love talking about your dolls, and the host today is Mary Beth. She'll help you too."

Mary Beth is the QVC host that I've worked with for almost eight years. Though I've done appearances with other capable hosts, she and I have a complimentary way of working together on air. I love her to pieces. We are like a couple of girlfriends, just shooting the breeze and having a blast. I always feel confident that it will be a good show when she is hosting. This information did make me feel calmer, but I was still having a hard time catching my breath.

Lisa stepped into the hallway and found Karl, who was waiting to walk me to the stage. He came into the dressing room and, seeing me curled up on the floor, thought the best thing he could do for us in that moment was to say a prayer to calm me. It worked. I was able to regain enough composure to go on.

The three of us walked down the hallway to the stage. Lisa pulled open the stage door and at the last moment said, "Did I mention that there's a live studio audience for today's show?"

I didn't even have time to react before she gently pushed me onto the set. I'm sure she thought that if I knew I was going to have three hundred doll fans in the audience it might push me over the top, and she was right. But she also knew that it would be the best thing for me. I found myself standing up straighter and genuinely smiling and responding to the outpouring of affection from the audience. One thing both Lisa and Karl know is that I love people and I really do find happiness in creating happiness for others. I did get through all the shows that day, but it took a lot of determination (and even more chocolate).

◆

When I got back to Los Angeles, I could no longer hold up under any pressure. I had found it almost impossible to get through a weekend of QVC shows, so the thought of returning to a daily talk show had me in a complete panic. I couldn't keep up any appearance of being okay, regardless of who was around me. I felt I had to isolate myself from my family and friends. I especially didn't want my kids to be afraid of me, but I didn't see how they couldn't be. I was afraid of me. I was afraid of what was happening to me. And now, since I had tried to go back to work, it was evident that no amount of willpower or attempts to change my attitude were making a difference. I was in a depression.

Accepting that this was true, I had to face my feelings about depression. I think I was afraid of a lack of self-control, so I had a narrow opinion of what depression was and wasn't. I was inclined to think that those suffering depression must not have known how to look at the good things in life, or that they were too focused on themselves. I was sure that discipline and hard work were cure-alls for almost everything, because they had always kicked me out of the blues in the past. I had determined that depression could be overcome as soon as one made the choice to put out the effort. Now depression had become my reality, and now I realized that choice had absolutely nothing to do with it. I was going to need help.

I placed a call to the physician who would have delivered my baby if I had been in Los Angeles. I described some of what I was going through while still trying to be cheerful (even in this circumstance!). He was kind and reassuring over the phone. He told me that many, many women experience a temporary depression following childbirth and said that a short-term prescription for an antidepressant would pull me out of it. He said he would call in the prescription, which I should try for five days and then call him back.

I have never had an issue with the idea of taking medication for any other condition. If you have to take a thyroid pill, high-blood-pressure medication, or allergy shots, then you do. If you need it, then you need it. But I was having a hard time with this one. I didn't want to admit that I needed an antidepressant. Wouldn't that mean I was incapable of functioning normally?

Despite my reluctance, I agreed to give it a try because it was obvious I really did need something to help me get through the day. I was hoping that what I was going through was as simple as what my doctor had described over the phone and that the answer was close at hand. In my heart, though, I knew it was more complicated than a temporary problem with the way the neurotransmitters were firing in my brain.

I know antidepressants have been successful in treating many women with PPD, but the one I was given wasn't the answer for me. It did help in lifting the severe lows, but it also took away my ability to feel any joy. No lows and no highs. I was robotic. I could function, but that was all.

I called the doctor back after the five days and described my experience on the antidepressant. He told me that every drug had some type of side effect and then asked me jokingly, "What do you want, the perfect drug?"

I laughed along and said, "Yes. Yes, I do." Little did he know how much I meant that.

In retrospect, I should have said, "The medication isn't working. What else can we try?" But I was feeling humiliated because I hadn't bounced back, I had let the doctor down. Again, I wasn't being a One-Take Osmond. I scolded myself for expecting too much and just quit taking the anti-depressant.

Two events took place during the week I was on the anti-depressant medicine. I have very little memory of either. The first was the day of Matthew's blessing at our church. This was a time for family and friends to gather in celebration of the new baby's being given a name and a blessing. The day of the blessing had always been joyful and significant for me with each of my other children. I remember sitting and holding Matthew during the service and looking at the faces of my children and my friends. They all had tears of joy in their eyes, but not me. I waited for the joy to overtake me, but I felt nothing. When I look at pictures of me taken that day, I can see what effect the antidepressant had on me. This should have been one of the happiest days in my life as a parent, but instead it was a flat line. My mouth is smiling in these pictures, but my eyes are vacant and empty, as if I'm not even there. I'll always regret the loss of feeling on a day that should have been a sweet and heartfelt memory.

The other occasion was a professional meeting with a new publicist, Marleah Leslie, who is well-known in Hollywood. Publicists help to coordinate a public figure's exposure in the press. They release statements for the celebrity when the press is seeking personal information, and they decide what one-on-one interviews should be given to which magazines or newspapers. They also release announcements of upcoming events, like albums, movies, and television appearances.

The day I was to meet with her, I was feeling totally numb. Karl and I were in my office at the *Donny & Marie* soundstage. He gave me my schedule for the day, starting with the meeting with Marleah. I told him that it was impossible for me to meet someone new because I felt like a zombie, and he assured me he would stick by me through the meeting and add to the conversation. During the interview, I just sat there in a black dress and dark glasses. I think I only nodded yes or no to Marleah's questions and shook her hand when she left. As soon as the door closed I asked Karl, "Do you think she could tell how out of it I am?"

Well, I'm often reminded how subjective perception is, and this incident is a prime example. Marleah called Karl soon after the interview, saying she was excited to work with me and had found me to be intelligent, serious, and full of creative thoughts. I have no idea how she arrived at that description. I was convinced following that interview that she was probably thinking something like, "If the studios ever decide to remake *The Stepford Wives,* Marie's our gal!"

14

"It's Donny and ... Who Is That?"

I'm not ready to come back to work" is probably the last thing the executive producers of a national television show want to hear from the host. We were scheduled to start production for the second season of *Donny & Marie* in five days, during the third week of August, and I was in their office, with Karl by my side, telling Charlie Cook and Maureen Fitz-Patrick that I wasn't sure I was able to do the show.

As I sat there trembling, trying to hold back my emotions, I said, "I think you need to know what I've been going through. I've been massively depressed." It was hard for me to tell them the whole story, but I knew I had to. Karl filled in some of the details of the prior few weeks for me and told them that I was concerned that emotionally, and maybe physically, I couldn't keep up with the rigorous schedule that comes with doing a talk show. I felt they should know that I wasn't myself and I wasn't sure when or if I would be again.

"I really don't know what's wrong, but I know there must be answers," I said, trying to convince myself as well.

Though they were sympathetic and encouraging, it was clear it would be impossible to postpone taping the show. We had to premiere the new season on schedule. The stations had been promised new shows, and everyone—production staff, crew, and guests—was ready to go. After the meeting, I knew I would have to find a way to pull it together enough to "stand and deliver," as they say. I would have to draw from every resource that had worked in the past: every trick, illusion, method, and discipline that helped me project an image on stage when I didn't feel as if I could face an audience. Since I wasn't myself, I would have to re-create the Marie Osmond that everyone expected to see.

My fatigue level seemed to be at an all-time high. Just managing to get through a regular day without any public appearances was a test of sheer willpower. I couldn't imagine where I would find the energy to do the show or the accompanying press interviews, photo sessions, and appearances that would resume in full force within days.

The first week of taping was uncomfortable in almost every way. My body felt foreign to me. I was still so achy, and I hated to be on TV when I could barely hide the dark circles under my eyes, my face was puffy, and I was carrying extra weight.

When I heard through the grapevine that the executives had made mention that I was still overweight, I was instantly flooded with painful memories of being criticized about my weight as a teenager. The same sting of humiliation that I had felt years before returned as strongly as if no time had passed at all. But this time there was a difference. I wasn't defeated by the hurt. It turned into anger. I was a thirty-nine-year-old woman who had given birth six weeks earlier. I thought it was an unrealistic expectation for me to be back to my pre-pregnancy figure. I didn't want to hear that I needed to lose weight; I knew that. I was already struggling with it every day, going through maddening times of trying to lose by depriving myself of food. Then I would feel so tired that I would end up quickly eating things that would provide an instant boost, usually carbohydrates and sugars.

The executives had also suggested that it was time to update my image for the new season. Part of that decision involved bringing in a new hairstylist and a new makeup person, despite my request to keep the ones I had. This was a very distressing change for me. I've never had a problem updating my image. I'm known for changing my hairstyle in a moment's notice. I've had them all. My problem was with the decision to not rehire the stylists I had worked with for many years of my career, Bob and Gail. They were both very talented and able to replicate any new look that the studios thought would be good for me to try. They knew every peculiarity of my hair and my skin and how to make the new look work for me. I felt safe with them. They knew my personality and had become dear and trusted friends over the years. With them I could show my emotions and talk about what I was going through. They had always protected my privacy. Having to acquaint myself with new people and teach them the techniques that worked best for me on camera meant one more thing for me to worry about. And it was painful to experiment with a new image when I was barely hanging on to the old one. I couldn't stand to look at myself.

When I learned that changes would be made regardless of my feelings, I tried to put it into the perspective of the show business world. I know I'm a commodity. I've always tried to separate Marie Osmond the entertainer from Marie the person. But, no matter how strongly I stated my reasons to rehire them as my stylists for season two, I felt that I was voiceless and that my title of executive producer was just a nod from the studio that held no authority.

My reflection in the mirror would stop me in my tracks.

I was unrecognizable to myself. It was like looking across a room full of people and seeing someone you think you know but being unsure of who it is. Every day the look on my face reminded me of news footage of people who have gone through a natural disaster, such as a hurricane or tornado, and return to find their homes leveled. It's the unbelieving look in their eyes when they say, "Everything I worked for is gone. I'll have to start over again. There's nothing else I can do." I felt so removed from my own face and body, I couldn't believe other people could recognize me.

I thought the show announcer was going to open the show any day now by saying, "From the Sony Studios in Los Angeles, California, it's Donny and . . . who is that?"

My disconnection from my physical self represented what I was feeling inside. I was having a difficult time finding my "stage legs" again. Every day I had to relearn my job. I felt as if I had lost my confidence and pacing as a host. The comfort level I had established by the end of the first season was gone. Nothing came back to me naturally. I couldn't quickly absorb necessary information the way I'd always been able to. I was afraid to go into the studio audience to shake hands after the shows because I thought audience members might see how miserable I was really feeling and that it might cause me to break down in tears. Talking about my life during the opening of the shows was almost torturous. I didn't feel funny or able to find the humor in almost any topic.

How could I find humor or laugh at myself when I couldn't even figure out who I was anymore? In the early morning, driving into the studio, I would ask myself: What was my identity now? Was I a mother? A performer? A talk show host? A wife? A woman? A businessperson? Would I ever be able to do any of these things well again?

A wax museum in Southern California had asked Donny and me if they could create our likenesses for display. We agreed, and they came to take our measurements and shoot rolls of photos, three hundred and sixty degrees around each of us, from head to foot. I found it ironic that I was going to be immortalized fat in wax. Then I thought, "Hey, why don't I offer to just go stand in the museum? After all, no one would know the difference." I had so much in common with a wax figure. I too was existing without a pulse. Why couldn't my wax figure be having a meltdown instead of me? Someday, I plan to sneak in there with a blowtorch and take off ten pounds.

My focus was so diminished by the depression I was in that I had to put more than twice the normal effort into learning the rundown for the day ahead. Nothing stayed with me. It got so severe that Karl started to tell me my schedule only one hour at a time or only one item at a time. For example, he would say, "At eight A.M. you have an interview for Lifetime's *Intimate Portraits*. After that, I'll fill you in on what you need to do at nine."

Not only was I questioning who I was and what I was doing, but there were days when I couldn't remember who other people were. Hosting a show with four or five new guests every day is challenging enough when you're on top of the game. If you're fuzzy brained, well . . . good luck.

One lapse in memory happened on a busy day when a last-minute interview with a well-known and respected personality was added to the show. The producers filled me in on the person, his history in television, and the show he was on now. Then we rolled tape. Early on, about a minute into the interview, I panicked when I realized that I couldn't remember what show he was promoting, or even what he had done in the past. That instantly eliminated many questions, for obvious reasons. Fortunately, it forced me to improvise and ask more personal and fun questions, and the guest started telling some great stories from his long career.

After every interview segment, we always took a photo with the guest. I thanked him, said good-bye, and then motioned Maureen over to me.

"That was a great interview," she congratulated me. "Really fun to watch."

I leaned over to her and whispered, "Who was that again?"

She almost fell on the floor from laughing. She put her arm around me and said, "You just did a twelve-minute interview, and I never for a minute guessed how lost you were." I guess my years of training paid off. When you're performing a live show and you miss a dance step or flub a line on stage, you can't let it stop you. You have to make it look intentional and not let the audience see you mentally hustling to get back in sync with the show.

During one show when I was on the country music circuit, I was performing in front of more than seventy thousand people at a fairground in the South. It was a muggy summer night, and my face was sweating, causing my makeup to run. During my first song, the intense humidity got to my fake eyelashes, causing one of them to peel off and land on my cheek. It's pretty hard to make that one look intentional. I just ripped the other one off, and on with the show. As if that weren't enough, I had been a mere minute on stage when thousands of bugs swarmed to join me in the spotlight. I've been told that bugs are actually a good source of protein. I hope so, because I'm sure I swallowed the equivalent of a side of beef before the end of the show. Flossing after every show became part of the routine with those outdoor concerts.

◆

Donny was a lifesaver for me more than once. The best part about working with a sibling is that you can be completely honest because they're family. They can't really say "Get lost." (Okay, maybe once or twice we've told each other to get lost, but not on the serious stuff.) I could tell Donny what I was going through, and though I'm sure he didn't completely understand, he was as supportive as he could be. As he has written in his own book, he's no stranger to anxiety. He still battles it occasionally. We have such a long history of working together that I think only the two of us can understand what we've gone through. We've always been able to tell when there's something going on with the other, whether we talk about it openly or not. We seldom had personal struggles on the same day, so one of us would always take the lead and cover for the other. There were many days in the early weeks of the second season when my hands would start to tremble while we waited for our entrance at the beginning of the show. I could feel my heart skipping in my chest and I'd say to Donny, "Please, help me. I don't know if I can go out on stage and do this show." He'd put his arm around me and say, "Don't worry about it, sis. Lean on me. We'll get through this one together."

I give Donny a hard time on stage by teasing him and setting him up for jokes. It's our chemistry. It's how we developed our relationship on stage. He'll play along with almost anything, and that's what makes it so much fun to work with him. Donny is a true performer; he is amazingly quick and will put his all into everything he does. I've shared the stage with many male performers who are very good at what they do, but I can honestly say (and not because he's my brother) that Donny is the most all-around talent I know. I've watched him keep pace with Tommy Tune in a dance routine he learned just fifteen minutes before the show, spontaneously sing harmony with Stevie Wonder, and jump into a boxing exercise or a martial-arts demonstration with Chuck Norris and be moving like an expert within minutes. He can even put on a pair of six-inch platform shoes and walk the stage like a pro. That's a little scary.

Donny has kept a large base of fans for almost thirty years because he is absolutely genuine in his appreciation of them and wants to give them the best. But outside of his considerable talent and stage presence, my brother is truly a good man. I don't say that lightly, because I believe what they say about good men. They're hard to find.

◆

Somehow Donny and I always did make it through those first shows, although more than once I would go backstage during the commercial break and have what I'll refer to as a three-minute meltdown. That means after two minutes and fifteen seconds I had to stop crying, wipe my eyes, powder the tear marks in my makeup, pull out the Visine, put on my smile, and get back out there!

On the outside, all seemed well. The show's ratings were on the rise, and everyone seemed to be back in the groove. But what a lesson in humility those first months were for me. What a change from the person I knew myself to be. I was talking on stage, but I wouldn't feel as if the voice were connected to me. I could feel myself smiling and hear myself asking questions, but it was not connected to anything inside of me. I was still existing very far back, behind my eyes. A whole other me was taking over internally, observing the paces I was putting myself through, waiting for the moment the guard could come down. I was operating in the world of light and fun, but I was sharing the spotlight with something much more menacing than a bunch of bugs this time.

I couldn't let myself sink into darkness. I had to rise to another huge occasion. Donny and I had been invited to host the seventy-ninth annual Miss America pageant, an event that had been on my schedule for many months. For us to be able to host the pageant we had to tape extra *Donny & Marie* shows early in the week to cover the time we would be in Atlantic City. I had mentally braced myself for the nonstop workweek I was obligated to get through. I found it ironic when Hurricane Floyd skirted Atlantic City just thirty-six hours before the pageant. We arrived to a city boarded up to prevent windows from shattering, and the famous boardwalk girded for the gale force winds and rain. The city was doing everything it could to protect its fun and inviting image, but because it sits right on the ocean, it was fragile and exposed to forces out of its control. It seemed to symbolize my own state of existence.

There were other issues that were causing unrest too: a hotel workers' strike and changes in the rules of the pageant to include, among other things, contestants who had been married and divorced. Perhaps there was something about my outlook on life that gave me an even drier sense of humor, but to make light of the controversy, I opened my mouth and the pageant by saying, "For the first time in history, Miss America is going to have to share her scholarship winnings fifty-fifty with her ex-husband." That's the quote that made the newspapers across the country. Let's just say I was surprised when they asked me to come back to host Miss America in 2000.

The Miss America pageant is a major production. Trying to coordinate the judges, the music, the choreography, and fifty-one anxious young women in a three-hour television program is an all-out effort. Donny and I had about twenty-four hours to make our part of it look professional. I pushed any thoughts of weariness out of my head. I couldn't allow myself a moment to pause or even allow my feelings to surface because I knew I wouldn't be able to get through if I did. There were lyrics to learn, choreography to practice, and interviews with the press. We were in such a time crunch, I found myself up until five-fifteen in the morning the day of the pageant, working on formulating the interview questions for the finalists. I don't know if it was lack of sleep or a symptom of the war going on within my body, but I was unable to focus my vision, both close up and far away. "Great," I thought. "First the brain can't focus and now the eyes. Why couldn't it be my taste buds? They never seem to lose any focus." I resorted to a pair of glasses to see the interview questions on stage and still had a difficult time reading the type. The show was broadcast to millions worldwide and thousands were there with us, watching in the convention hall. I think it was thousands; it was all a big blur to me.

Being around fifty-one young and enterprising college women who didn't need glasses and who were looking forward to the choices and possibilities that their futures held filled me with an increasing sense of defeat about the possibility of ever feeling enthusiasm or hope again in my own life.

When I got on the plane to go back to California, I looked at my schedule for the next week. In twenty hours I was due back at the studio. With the exception of the baby, whom I took to Atlantic City with me, I hadn't seen my children in four and a half days. They were spending more time with nannies than their own mother. I knew that with all my professional obligations, my priorities had been shuffled and, to my great sorrow, my highest priority, my children, had ended up near the bottom of the list. I would be getting home in time to kiss them good-night and would leave early the next morning for the studio, so it wasn't as if I would be spending time with them when I got home. I was continuing to fail them. On the flight I read some articles I wanted to catch up on. One was a parenting article that stated that the maximum length of time a child should be separated from his or her mother is one day for each year of life. Meaning a two-year-old should not spend more than two consecutive days away from her mother, etc. My vision began to blur again, making it impossible to read. I reached up to rub my eyes and found the reason for the blurred vision. Tears. Yes, I was supporting my family. Yes, I was fulfilling my obligations. I was getting by. But what did getting by mean to my children? I knew I hadn't had seven children to let them be raised by others. Was I trying to be too much for too many at the expense of my children? This wasn't a flubbed line or a missed dance step. It was bigger than that. I felt the lasting bonds between a mother and her children were at stake. No amount of crying could relieve that deep a heartache.

◆

Starting the next day at the studio and continuing through the week, I would hold it together only until the end of the taping for the day and then get in my car to go home to my children. Almost every night as I drove, I would fall apart emotionally, deluged with guilt about the mother I wasn't capable of being anymore. The car was the one place I still had the privacy to let my feelings out.

One evening, I parked in the driveway, but I couldn't pull myself together enough to go into the house. I had been sitting in the car for about fifteen minutes when Brian discovered me. He came out to the car, opened the door, and urged me to come in the house to kiss my children good-night. I told him I couldn't let them see me so upset. He reminded me that the kids loved their mom and told me they would be okay with seeing my tears. I walked in with Brian but went straight up to bed because I was too uncomfortable with having the children see me cry so much.

There is an innocent wisdom in small children. One by one, my children came into the bedroom to be with me, which is what I needed the most. Brianna kissed my cheek sweetly and cuddled her face into my shoulder, and Brandon wrapped his little arms around my neck and said, "Don't cry, Mommy." Jessica and Rachael hugged me and curled up on the bed, and Michael squeezed in where he could to get close to me. Stephen took my hand in his and said, "We love you, Mom."

My children were and continue to be a respite in the storm, the reinforcement that kept my sense of self from shattering completely. Having them snuggle up against me was unbelievably comforting. It was the grace that only comes from unconditional love, which children give freely and unself-consciously. I wanted to stay there forever, surrounded by my sweet babies. I have always thought my daily mission as a mother was to keep my children safe, but in simple truth, they were forming a raft of love around me, keeping me afloat on my dark sea.

15

$\diamond$

A Whole Other Reality

If there were lessons to be learned from my postpartum depression, then pain was my teacher and it didn't appear I would graduate any time soon. Every day there were new lessons from a demanding instructor who held me in class until I stopped ignoring my need for help.

As soon as I started to feel as though the worst was behind me and I was going to be okay, an unexpected test would present itself. One I couldn't prepare for. There were hours of the day when I felt fine, close to being human, and then the depression would catch up with me. It would start out as a foggy feeling, then the darkness would begin to close in, and an emotional whirlwind would stir, slowly at first, then speeding, tossing my feelings around chaotically. It was like that game show in which the contestant steps into a glass booth and paper money is blown all around him. He tries to grab as much money as possible out of the frenzy before the wind dies down and the game is over. During this time, I felt as if everything I valued and believed about myself were being blown loose. All the deeply held images and labels and self-definitions were dragged up and put outside of me, where I could see them for what they were. Out of panic, I would grab for them and try to put them back so they couldn't get away again. I would scramble to save anything I could until I was left tired and empty. The torrent of emotions could last for an hour or sometimes the whole day, then leave me flattened, unable to move. Each time, I would recover and think that I had made it through the worst, until the next episode, when I would again struggle to hang on to the only me I knew, and in doing so, put an even deeper gouge in my injured sense of self.

I look back at those horrible days and weeks and ask, Why? Why did I allow this to continue? Why didn't I seek help? Why didn't I find a counselor? Why didn't I go to my doctor again? Why didn't I get a second opinion about other antidepressants I could try? Of course, these are all legitimate questions. I can say that if I had been watching a friend go through this experience, I would have asked the same questions. Questions like: What's wrong with her? There are resources a phone call away. Why doesn't she help herself? These are logical questions, based on good common sense and easily asked by a person in her right mind.

This is where depression is most harsh. I was not in my right mind. The depression had shut down all my extra mental and physical resources, leaving only those needed for basic survival. (And sadly, in some cases it robs people of their survival instincts as well.) Even though my mind was rarely at rest, I couldn't collect my thoughts enough to follow through on the steps it would have taken to get help. It's not easy to explain, but the idea of making a phone call, getting one more appointment in my hectic schedule, and then showing up for it and being able to tell the doctor what was going on with me was overwhelming. It was as impossible for me as if a surgeon said, "You're having an appendicitis attack," then handed me the scalpel and added, "Here you go. Have at it." Every bit of energy I had went into making sure my husband and kids were okay or doing the show. Almost everything else, including my relationships with my friends and my extended family, fell by the wayside. It was a combination of not having anything to spare and a feeling of deep shame at not being able to pull myself together. After all, it wasn't like appendicitis. No one's going to tell you to "snap out of it" when you are having an appendicitis attack.

Even though I was trying to convince everyone, myself included, that I was on an upward swing, it was always just a temporary feeling that would peak and then the gravity of depression would take effect again.

Shortly after returning from the Miss America pageant, I was scheduled to do an interview with a reporter from *TV Guide*, Mary Murphy. She wanted to talk about the return of the show and the birth of the baby. I was extremely hesitant to do an in-depth interview because I was not feeling mentally sharp. I talked for over an hour the morning of the interview to my executive producers, Charlie and Maureen, my publicist, Marleah, and my manager, Karl.

They all agreed it would probably be significant to women viewers if I let them know that I was having a bad case of baby blues. I wanted to be as honest as I could about what I was going through, without breaching my family's privacy, and let everyone know that I was trying to cope. It was becoming obvious to viewers who e-mailed or sent letters to the show that I wasn't my usual self, and I wanted to explain what was going on before the rumor mill turned it into something it wasn't.

I made it clear to Mary Murphy that I was only telling her about this in hopes that it would help other women realize they weren't alone. She acknowledged that she understood my purpose for giving the interview.

I've been around and involved in television for most of my life. I understand and can appreciate that network and cable shows are in constant competition to win viewers for their programs. An effective way for them to do this is through teases, which are exactly what the word sounds like. They tease you into watching with one little intriguing piece of the story, which keeps you tuned in to hear the rest. So when the *TV Guide* article was being promoted before it ran, of course the media featured the most sensational part of my interview—my drive up the coast. The promos made it sound as if I had walked out on my husband and abandoned my children without a word. The reality of the situation was completely downplayed: My children had been in our home, in capable adult hands, with access to anything they might have needed and access to their father.

Once the story broke, the tabloid newspapers and gossip shows began a feeding frenzy on my life. They followed me home from the studio and took unauthorized photographs of me with my children in our private lives. Any chance they could, they created story after story about my supposedly nasty behavior on the set and ran them along with photographs that were obviously from the 1980s. Photographs of me wincing in the sunlight, sneezing, or something equally attractive. I guess they wanted me to look as if I was in pain. (It was painful enough to look at the hairstyles I wore in those days.)

The *TV Guide* interview, with my description of what happened, didn't hit the stands until the week of November 13, which was four full weeks after the coastal drive was revealed on television. I did talk about my depression on *Donny & Marie* shortly after that, but it went somewhat unrecognized by the press. In the entertainment world, the bitter truth is often that no one wants to hear the truth. I'm well aware that every celebrity falls prey to unbridled gossip at some point. And I believe that the truth of every situation surfaces and expels bad or negative gossip eventually, but it was stressful for me to think of my older children being exposed to rumors and hurtful comments at school. Being the children of a public person had great perks for them, like travel and invitations to exciting events, but the downside was being exposed to public opinions about their parent and sometimes being talked about themselves.

Between the way I was feeling and the stress of having my drive up the coast reported in such a sensationalistic manner, I felt shook up from the inside out. I couldn't sit still at all: My legs would involuntarily bounce up and down as if an electrical current were shooting through them, my hands trembled, and on the inside I felt as though someone were tapping on my nerve endings with a steel hammer. Sleep was nearly nonexistent. I felt grateful if I could rest for two consecutive hours. I would lie down, but the shaking I felt inside made rest impossible. I had to get up and move. I would walk the floor most of the night, or read information and watch videos to prepare for the next day's show.

I was so upset that I was letting almost everything slip. I wasn't even able to wash my stage makeup off at the end of the day or comb through my hair. I didn't have the energy to do much more than brush my teeth. I would usually drop from complete fatigue at about four in the morning and have to get back up at six A.M. to leave. Brian had to drive me to the studio a handful of times because I couldn't keep my eyes open. Once I was at the studio, I would wash off the previous day's makeup, shampoo my hair, and start the whole process again.

One morning my hairstylist on the show started to work

on my hair, and the comb got caught up in a snag. Or at least we thought it was a snag.

"What in the world is this?" she asked leaning closer to my head to inspect the snarled section.

I put my hand up to my hair. I couldn't imagine what might be growing out of my head and I was scared to find out. Well, it wasn't something growing out of my head, it was something glowing on my head. A full-sized neon-colored gummy worm candy was matted in my hair. My kids had been sharing a bag of gummy worms while sitting on my bed the night before to watch a video, and one must have strayed . . . or been deliberately placed on my pillow. The fact that I could get up and leave with a four-inch lime green night crawler stuck to the back of my head shows just how oblivious I was to the way I looked. I had to laugh about it. What if someone else had spotted it? I guess I would have pretended it was a new fashion trend. At least gummy worms come in a variety of colors to match any outfit.

One afternoon, the sensation of my nerves being hammered on was so intense I felt as if I wanted to come right out of my own skin. Dina, my good friend and head of wardrobe for the show, brought in my outfit for the second show of the day, but I couldn't change clothes.

"Something is really wrong with me, Dina," I said. "I'm scared. I don't know what's happening, but I definitely feel ill, like my body is dying."

Dina wanted me to go to the doctor right then, but I knew I had to make it through the next show as usual. I couldn't call it quits and leave everyone hanging. I made it through the show, but I was sure that what I was feeling on the inside must be showing on the outside because it was so extreme. I thought it had to be noticeable that my nerves were rattling around under my skin. At one point, I did almost give in and leave the stage.

Sometimes surrender is exactly what's called for. That night I felt like a caged animal, caged in my own body. I couldn't sleep or even lie down. The house felt like a trap to me. At three in the morning, I pulled on my robe and went out to walk the neighborhood. Each house was dark and silent; all of my neighbors seemed to be sleeping peacefully. I looked at the surrounding hills, the moon, and the stars. I knew nearby, in the brush behind the houses, were probably skunks, coyotes, deer, possums, and owls, a whole other world that operates on a different schedule from that of humans. During these hours the neighborhood belonged to them. Theirs was a whole other reality, a valid existence that I rarely experienced, and that made me think about what was going on with me. The fact that I had never experienced such a severe depression before didn't mean it wasn't a reality for me right now. I was existing in the dark, even though it wasn't a natural place for me to be. I decided it was time to accept that this was where I was and surrender my battle against myself. I knew I couldn't just bandage the experience and make it better. I was wounded and I needed help. I sat down on the curb and dropped my head into my hands and prayed, "I submit myself to you. I can't do it. Please intercede in my life. Not my will, but Yours."

I believe that prayer is much more than consolation of the heart. Thought is energy and I believe it's actual communication with God. I think He expects us to help ourselves, but in those moments of despair when a solution can't be found, I try to be still and listen for a prompting that helps me know His will. Often the briefest of prayers will help me trust that I will find guidance and an answer that is always beyond my personal wisdom.

The next morning, the heaviness had lifted enough for me to think about where I could go for help. I strongly felt that I had to find someone I could trust and not feel hesitant to talk with. I needed a doctor with whom I didn't feel obligated to put on the smile. I didn't want to be diagnosed with the baby blues. I'd had the baby blues before following my other births, and this wasn't it. This was much darker than blue. I remembered Dr. Judith Moore, in Utah. She was a doctor my mother-in-law had told me about when I was suffering through a persistent case of mono. Judith had helped me regain my energy through natural means, and I wondered if she could help me again. I have always responded well to natural healing techniques, which she emphasized in her practice. I felt instinctually that she would have some answers, but her practice was in Provo, Utah, and my chances of leaving L.A. at that time were slim. I made the call anyway and told her that something was severely off in my system but that I wouldn't be able to come to her office for at least three weeks. She explained how a number of factors, including hormone imbalances, could trigger a postnatal reaction, and that the symptoms I was describing to her indicated that I was suffering from postpartum depression. She explained to me in clear terms why this was much more than the baby blues and said we should start with some blood work right away. She told me I could have the tests done in L.A. and the results sent to her. She would be able to study the reports to see what was happening. She ordered a variety of tests. (Please refer to Dr. Moore's section at the end of the book for a description of available blood tests.) My schedule was jammed, and I wasn't sure how I would find the time to get to the doctor's office, but I knew I had to help myself. And I think this was one of those times I needed to move Heaven and Earth to get it done.

My doctor in L.A., after seeing the results of the blood work, called me at home the next day. He said my estrogen was very low, so he called in a prescription for Premarin, which I was to start taking that very day.

I thought I was starting to find some answers. Gaining any insight into my condition helped me feel more stable than I had in weeks. It turned out to be a short-lived recess from my anxiety, because I had a severe reaction to the Premarin the next day at work.

It was a day we were taping two shows back to back. Near the end of the first show, I started to get a severe headache, which led to nausea. I tried to lie down for a short time between shows, but my heart started racing and I felt short of breath. I wasn't sure what was going on, but it was frightening, to say the least. Karl and my assistant on the show, Missy Garcia, tried to calm me and talk me through the pain. I tried taking ibuprofen and putting a cold pack on my eyes. Nothing worked. The headache wasn't letting up at all. I thought it might be the onset of a migraine, because I'd had them before, but this one felt different. It wasn't a localized pain. My whole head felt ready to explode. I had less than a half hour before the next show was scheduled to start, and I couldn't keep my eyes open because of the pain. Karl told the executive producers of my condition, and they debated whether or not to get someone to fill in for me. They thought a doctor should be called to my dressing room to check on me.

I told them, "No. As long as I can stand up and walk, I'm going to do the show. I'll get through this. Just give me a little time." Once everyone was out of the dressing room, I had Missy call Dr. Judith. She wasn't at her office, but someone managed to track her down and she soon called back. She thought I was having a reaction to the estrogen and that it would pass. She talked me through an acupressure technique she used on patients in her office. She encouraged me and advised me step by step how to release whatever was making matters worse. Her voice was so calm and reassuring over the phone that within minutes my heart slowed and my nausea eased up. After a short period of time my headache became tolerable. There are many stories of mind over matter, but I'm always amazed at the close relationship between the mind and the body. Talking to Dr. Judith in those minutes reversed the chain reaction of pain and panic that was going on in my body. I felt like a different person within twenty minutes.

When Karl saw me again after the phone call, he couldn't believe how much better I looked. He just shook his head and said, "I don't know how she helped you that much over the phone, but we should bottle and sell it." I believe Dr. Judith helped me the most that day with her ability to reassure me that someone was there who could help me, that what I was experiencing was real but it could be handled, and that I wasn't losing my mind. She helped me feel strong again. This hope was a liaison to my healing.

◆

I try to teach my kids that though the bad stuff looms large at times, there is always plenty of good to counterbalance it if you just look for it. I was reminded of this myself in many ways while going through this rough time in my life. So many dear fans sent me notes and e-mails of encouragement and understanding. My peers in the business were also wonderfully sympathetic and supportive. Kathie Lee Gifford sent me many thoughtful notes over three or four months, a gesture I will always remember. Whoopi Goldberg sent over a mammoth basket of bath products with a card saying, "Just because I love you." Garth Brooks left a message on my voice mail expressing concern and a willingness to help any way he could. Billy Joel sent a lovely note via Donny. Wynonna Judd called several times. Many other entertainers I had become friends with over the years left messages or sent notes. Celebrities are often categorized as self-involved and even arrogant. There are a few of those, but thankfully there are more kindhearted, generous people in this business than not, and I've been fortunate to meet and work with many of them.

I was reminded daily of the angels in human form all around me by the small and not-so-small acts of kindness they performed for me. My neighbor Mike would bring over homemade meatballs for dinner. Marcia, our head writer, gave me hand and neck massages that saved my life! My treasured assistant on the show, Missy, kept me organized, read me jokes from the Internet, and made sure I ate nutritious meals. Every day during the briefing for the shows, the hardworking producers, the writers, and Donny and I would cut up and goof around for at least thirty minutes. I've never met people who loved to laugh more than this group. Their humor was more healing to me every day than any medication I had tried. The crew was always nearby with smiles and words of encouragement. Guests who appeared on our show would often comment to me on the familylike atmosphere. The staff made every guest feel so special, they all wanted to come back again, from Jennifer Love Hewitt to Kirk Douglas.

There were also the angels unaware, as they say. There was the stranger in the next car on the highway who put on his brakes, smiled, and waved me into bumper-to-bumper traffic. There was the woman who spotted me in the checkout lane at the grocery store and, as she wheeled her cart out the door, caught my eye and mouthed the words "I love you." Every day, one moment of interaction would cut through the darkness and I would remember that life is good and sorrow is temporary, and that through sorrow we can respect and appreciate joy. I began to open my eyes to what the pain had to teach me and how I could use what I was learning. That's when a call came in from Oprah.

16

◆

The Larger Picture

"You gain strength, courage and confidence by every experience in which you really stop to look fear in the face."

—ELEANOR ROOSEVELT

Oprah wanted me to come on her show and talk about postpartum depression. My first response was "No, but thank you anyway." I had talked publicly about it once already and the slanted way the tabloids and others in the media had handled it made me want to avoid doing it again. I wasn't an expert on postpartum depression, in fact, I was just learning about it myself and felt I was barely on the other side of my own darkest moments. I didn't think I should be looked to for an answer. I called Charlie Cook, our executive producer, and told him I didn't feel comfortable about doing Oprah's show.

He reminded me that it would be a chance to tell my story not through the media's interpretation but in my own voice to millions of people. He said that I didn't have to be the expert, that my own experiences were enough.

I told him I would give it more thought over the weekend. I wasn't at all interested in exposing my children to more public opinion about their mother's problems. Those opinions were already following them home from school in the form of comments like "What's up with your mom? I heard she's psycho." I just wanted to find some answers, get through it, and never look back. So why would I want to recount it all on *Oprah*? There wasn't one logical reason. But, as well I know, the heart isn't logical.

I kept reflecting on how much my mother had helped me through my lowest hours with that phone call in the motel room. I had often wondered where I would be if she had not shared her story with me. It had sparked a flame, and however dim it was in some moments, it was a beginning. I held on to her story with hope for my own future. During the weekend, I started feeling something completely different than I expected. I no longer cared about setting the record straight on why I drove up the coast. It wasn't about that anymore. I felt I was being guided to an objective much larger than my own recovery. I had to say yes.

A date was set for me to do *Oprah*, but apprehension about appearing began to grow daily. After all, wouldn't they have the right to point a finger at me and ask all those questions I had asked myself: Why didn't I get help? I had enough money; why didn't I take care of myself? What about all the women who couldn't leave their kids with a babysitter and get away?

I had no idea what I'd say or how to begin describing what I was going through, but I thought that if I could just be honest about what it was like for me, then perhaps it would help another woman describe it to her doctor, or husband, or children.

The Osmonds have never been ones to "air their dirty laundry," as my parents would put it. They raised us to believe that our family had received so many blessings (and we have), that to disclose personal problems was thoughtless. They would remind us that no matter what we were going through, someone else was going through much more, "so we should be grateful for our problems and not complain."

When I called to tell my mother what I had decided to do, she voiced her concern about how it would be perceived.

"Mother," I replied, "do you know what you did to help me? You made me feel I wasn't alone in the world and going crazy. I had put all of that stress on myself, that I was incapable of handling seven children and yet you had raised nine. Then I got to see a part of you that I didn't know about, one brief period of time when you couldn't handle it either. You gave me the strength to get through it. You did, so I knew I could. Maybe by talking about it, I could do that for another woman."

"I just don't know if I want the world to know I went through it," my mother admitted.

I knew that by telling my story I couldn't avoid telling hers. I tried to be considerate of what that would mean to her, but her reservations also confirmed for me how much postpartum depression needed to be talked about. Here was my mother, who in my eyes was the perfect idea of a woman, feeling self-conscious about a natural experience she had gone through thirty-seven years before. Seeing that she was still feeling embarrassment about it made it clear to me that the issue of postpartum depression had been hidden away for too long. I understood, though, because I had similar feelings about it myself. I didn't want to become the face connected with postpartum depression. Still, I knew in my heart that I might help others by telling my story, and in the end, that's what had made me say yes to Oprah.

Oprah Winfrey has probably done more than any other talk show host in history to enlighten the public on issues

My mother and my daughter Rachael. I got my smile from my mother. She got her gray streaks from me. (*Osmond Family Archive*)

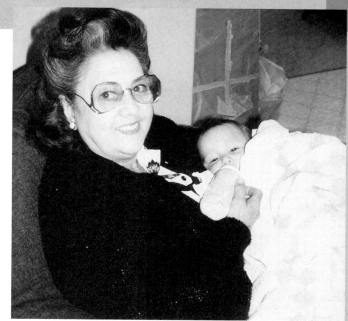

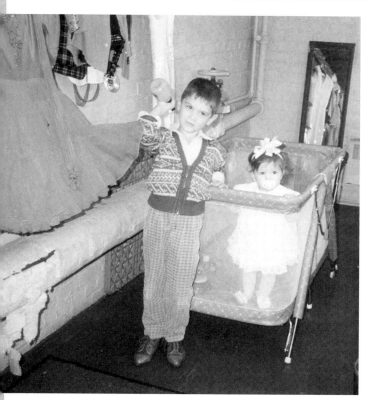

The world is a stage but my world was in my dressing room. My babies, Stephen and Jessica. (*Osmond Family Archive*)

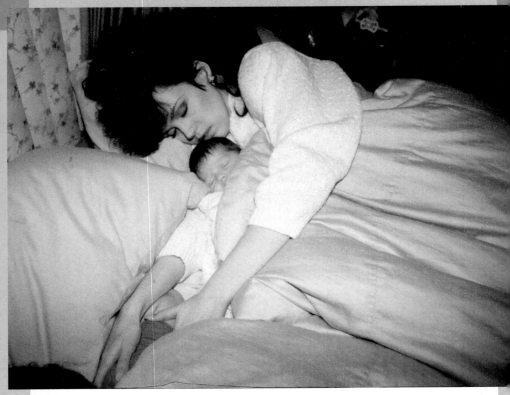

Grabbing forty winks on the road with Jessica.
(*Osmond Family Archive*)

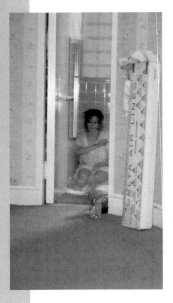

This is where you could find me in between shows while touring. An endless bout of mono made having a normal diet impossible—my body rejected it all. My kids took this glamor shot of Mom. (*Osmond Family Archive*)

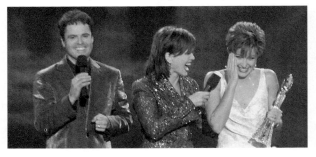

Donny and I present Miss America 2000, Heather French, with the Woman of Achievement Award. The Miss America Doll I created was actually designed to capture Heather's beauty and charm. (*Photo courtesy of the Miss America Organization*)

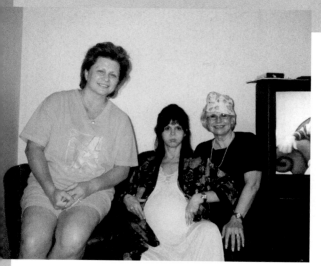

Back home after twenty hours of labor and no baby. My friend Patty and my mother-in-law Georgia Blosil came by to cheer me up. I can't believe I'm putting this photo in my book! (*Osmond Family Archive*)

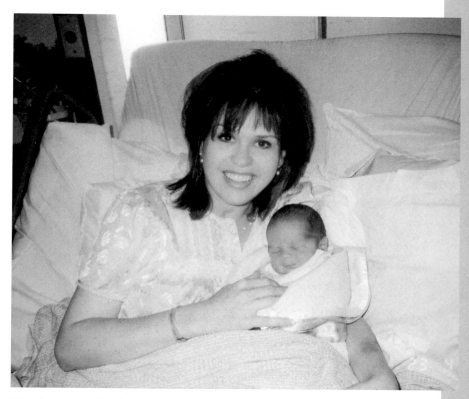

Matthew R. Blosil, one day old. All I wanted to do is take a long nap with my baby. (*Osmond Family Archive*)

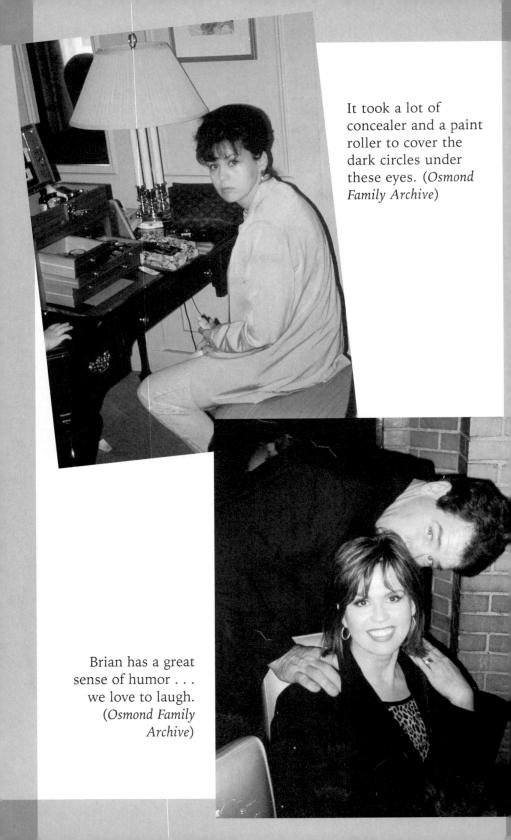

It took a lot of concealer and a paint roller to cover the dark circles under these eyes. (*Osmond Family Archive*)

Brian has a great sense of humor . . . we love to laugh. (*Osmond Family Archive*)

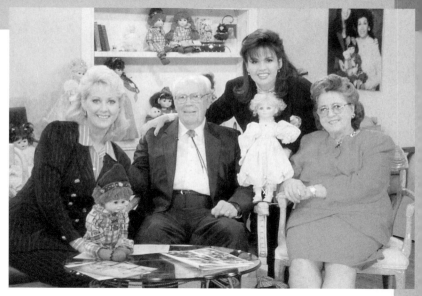

The "Show" always went on . . . my friend and QVC co-host, Mary Beth, along with my father, mother, and Georgette, my father's first sculpted doll. (*Osmond Family Archive*)

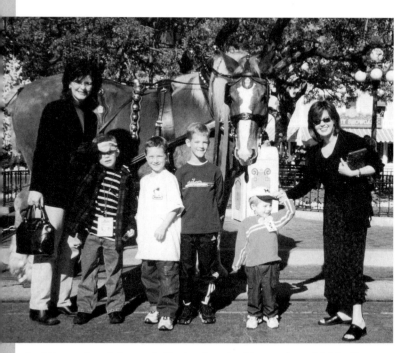

At Disneyland for a doll signing in December 1999. From left to right, Lisa Hatch, Lisa's son Drew, my son Michael, my nephew Nicholas, my son Brandon, and myself. (*Osmond Family Archive*)

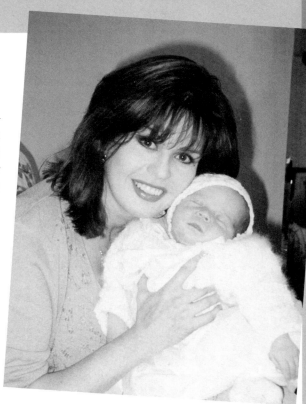

Baby Matthew—
one month old on
his blessing day!
(*Osmond Family
Archive*)

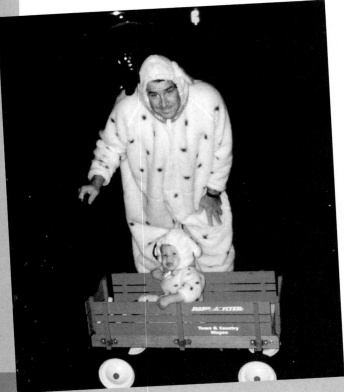

Brian and Matthew—
pretty cute pups
howling at the moon
on Halloween night.
(*Osmond Family
Archive*)

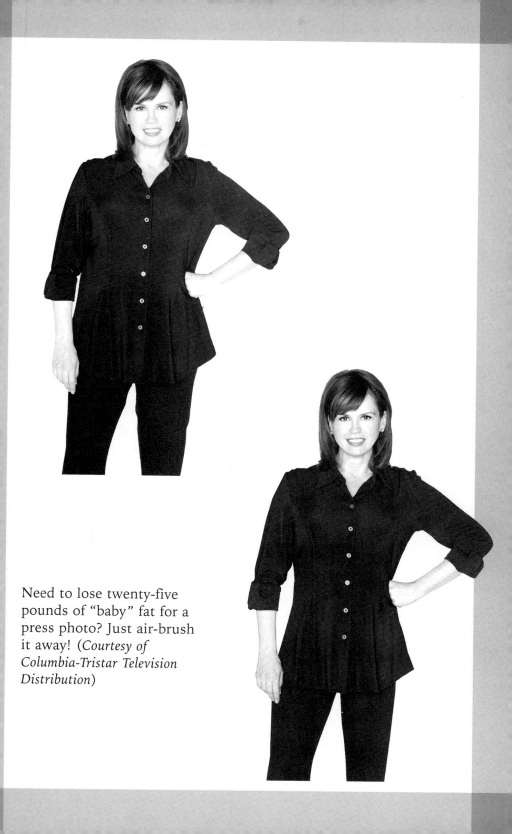

Need to lose twenty-five pounds of "baby" fat for a press photo? Just air-brush it away! (*Courtesy of Columbia-Tristar Television Distribution*)

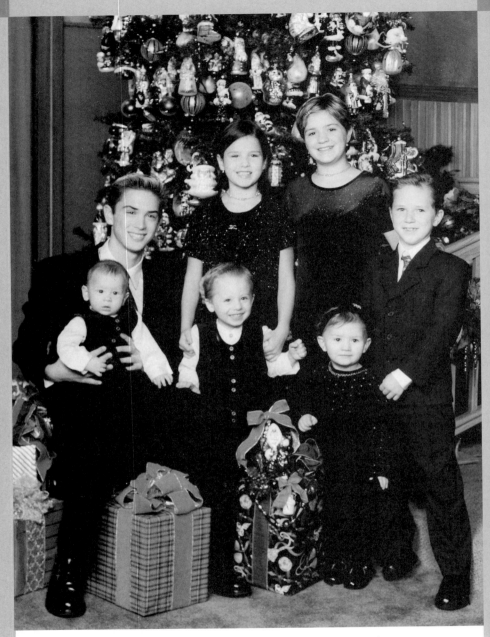

Christmas 1999. The best gifts I've ever received—my children. From left to right, Stephen with Matthew, Rachael with Brandon, Jessica, Brianna, and Michael. (*Photo by Merrett Smith*)

that women face daily. For many women, she is a sage, bringing them new information and knowledge to benefit their lives. Fortunately for her vast audience, Oprah has merited the authority to present subject matters she feels are important to women, and though postpartum depression affects only about 15 percent of all women who give birth, she still saw it as important enough to fill an hour-long show.

The morning of the show I was feeling uneasy and shaky from crying most of the night before. I had never publicly said much about my personal life, and now, feeling as bad as I did, it seemed hard to believe I was going to start here. I wanted to disappear. My *TV Guide* article had still not been published, so the only things most of this audience would have read or heard were the most sensational parts of my story. I was apprehensive about how they would receive me. I wondered if an audience of mothers might judge me harshly and be reluctant to understand how I could be depressed with all that my life offered. I was still not feeling like myself and I had reservations about my ability to answer tough questions, but I had to trust my reason for doing the show.

When I walked out on stage, the women in the audience embodied that reason. As I told my story, I looked out at the faces and saw women nodding their heads in understanding or sympathy. It was like a gathering of women who had traveled alone for a long time, feeling foreign to themselves, finally meeting others who shared their language. I felt at that moment that everyone in the room knew my pain. We related and shared empathy, understanding, and ultimately hope. I felt as if we all belonged to an elite group . . . the PPD club. The sorority no one chooses to rush.

During one of the commercial breaks I spoke with an audience member who sat crying in the front row, next to her husband. She could barely speak to me. I recognized the pain in her eyes, the loss of hope and the emotional frailty that had taken over her daily existence due to PPD. It was a despair of the deepest kind. I knew, because it was the look I saw in my own eyes every day.

I took her hand for a moment and all I could say was, "I know where you are. I understand."

"You give me hope that I can survive," she told me.

I wanted her to believe that there was help for her. I wanted to believe there was help for me. I don't often use the word *promise* because it's difficult to guarantee the outcome of almost anything. So I surprised myself when I said to the young woman, "I promise that you'll get better. I know there are answers."

Before I left her to go back on stage she said, "I'm holding you to that promise."

It was fascinating to hear the stories of other women unfold, and to witness the support for each woman from the audience as a whole. At the end of the show that day, I told the audience how touched I was by the experience. I also told them that I was going to search for some answers, and that when I found solutions I wouldn't keep them a secret.

Following the taping, Karl and Charlie, who had come to Chicago with me, told me it had been a good show and that they suspected I must be exhausted. Instead, the energy from the audience and the release that had come with discussing PPD with other women had actually been invigorating. I felt the good type of tired, but nothing revives me faster than shopping.

I grabbed Karl and Charlie by the arms: "What? Are you kidding? We're in Chicago, the home of Marshall Field's department store! Come on. Let's shop till we drop, or at least until we have to catch our flight back to L.A."

Suddenly I became Air Osmond, soaring down Michigan

Avenue, scoring some fabulous markdown purchases, and slam-dunking Frango Mints, a Chicago specialty, before Karl and Charlie could even raise their arms in defense.

The next day, when I arrived at the *Donny & Marie* studio, Missy brought a stack of papers into my dressing room.

"What's all of this?" I asked her.

"This is just some of all the e-mails you've received about your appearance on *Oprah* yesterday," she informed me.

I looked through them. I was holding in my hands e-mails representing the lives of women across the United States. They were thanking me for talking about my experience with PPD. It's rare for people to actually hear about how they may have affected someone else's life. Each of the stories was different, but they all made a reference in some way to one thing we shared: shame. Shame that had caused them to remain silent about their problem. Many of their messages said that it helped them so much just to know they weren't the only ones who were suffering. They pleaded with me to keep searching for answers.

Over the course of the next week, thousands of e-mails and handwritten letters came in about postpartum depression. My friend Lisa called from my Utah office to say that hundreds were also coming in from my doll collectors. As gratifying as it was to know that the *Oprah* appearance had touched so many women in a personal way, as I suspected, there was little positive news on how they were being helped. I had told my story, but the truth was I didn't even know how to help myself. I had now personally heard from thousands of women who were suffering in silence. If all of these women had taken the time and energy to write, how many more were there? Perhaps my part in it represented one small step in breaking the silence, but where were the answers?

After reading many letters, I realized that the very first step to healing was to somehow dispel the shame women feel for being depressed. There is no reason to feel shame. I believe that women are the life force, not only because we can have children, but also because of how we take care of the world. We are the nucleus of life, home, and family.

I thought about the wonderful qualities of the women I know. They serve as Scout leaders, child-care workers, PTA members, coaches, Sunday school teachers, and tutors. They are loyal to their families and friends. They take food to their housebound neighbors. They volunteer for charitable organizations. They go to any length to help their children excel. They voice their concerns about injustice and rally to pass laws to protect the helpless. They supply library books for the branch in the low-income neighborhoods. They go to the doctor with someone who's afraid. They stay up until two A.M. to help their teenager with a term paper and get back up at six to make breakfast, in many cases before they start their nine-to-five jobs. They bring happiness and hope, compassion and solutions.

It seems to me that women, who are so good at finding solutions for other people's problems, would have tremendous power if we would acknowledge our own needs as well, giving us self-worth.

I was a woman with postpartum depression. The response to my appearance on *Oprah* told me there were thousands of others. If, as individuals, we could begin to count ourselves as important, then together we had a strong chance of finding some solutions. I called Dr. Judith Moore. "I'm coming in," I said. "It's time to take care of myself."

17

A Verdict of Not Guilty

My son Stephen has a lightning-fast mind and a take on life that is almost always entertaining. A number of years ago, he was sent to his room as punishment for an episode of lying. I try to impress on my kids that it's one thing to do something wrong, but it's even worse to lie about it, because then it becomes a matter of trust. So usually my children will just tell me what they've done wrong, even before I hear what happened. They know I'm much easier on them when they take responsibility for what they've done, so it's a lot less stressful for them in the long run to 'fess up in the short. I make it so easy for them to tell me the truth that I'm surprised the confessions haven't started coming before the crimes: "Mom, in about an hour, I'll be playing outside when I'm supposed to be practicing piano. Just thought you should know."

I don't expect my kids to uphold any rules that I break myself, so I made Stephen look me in the eyes and I said, "Stephen, I'll never lie to you." He looked at the floor, brushed his hand across his mouth, faked a cough, and mumbled, "Santa Claus." I had to admit, he almost had me on that one. I did manage to recover and respond by saying, "That wasn't a lie. There truly was a Santa Claus and others have continued to carry his good works forward." Aren't I quick?

Explaining to a child the difference between a harmful lie and a fun tradition is not easy. I mean, there couldn't be any harm in having a child believe that his good behavior would be rewarded by a jolly man in a red suit with the toys that he's wished for all year. Or maybe there could. When I considered the Santa Claus principle, that good is rewarded with good and bad brings on bad, in light of my depression, it made me contemplate the ways this early belief may affect us as adults. If this rule of behavior was true, then how did it apply to what I was going through right now and what I had been through as a child? Hadn't it proved to be false in my own life? What I desired most was to be a good mother and wife, so why had I been rewarded with depression?

I believe this is why it's so difficult for women experiencing PPD, or any kind of depression, to talk to their doctors or anyone about it candidly. I know my feelings of inadequacy and embarrassment at not being able to cope caused me to downplay my true condition to my doctor, my neighbors, my coworkers, my extended family, and eventually even to myself. I was also afraid of hearing that it was all in my head. Instead of suffering the possible humiliation it might take to get help, I convinced myself that if I could find a way to control it by giving a little more, pushing myself further, and making it through one more day, then I would get better because I was trying harder.

Santa was obviously not going to make an appearance and give me what I was wishing for. I was going to have to search it out, pay for it, wrap it up with a big bow, and put my own name on the tag before I could have the package that held the answer for me. It was something I needed to give myself, not something to please my kids, my husband, my friends, or my coworkers. This had to be something I wanted.

◆

Dr. Judith Moore has raised six children of her own and began studying medicine when the youngest was a preschooler. Though she is a doctor of osteopathy, she has always studied natural healing techniques.

I felt so comfortable at my first appointment, I decided to tell her the whole truth about what I was going through both physically and emotionally. I described it all: feeling weepy, my muscle spasms, anxiety attacks, self-anger, and even my retreat to the closet floor and drive up the coast. I described how hard it was for me to even get out of bed and how much I cried. I told her of my heartaches and my hopelessness. She listened to it all with real interest and, I felt, without judgment. Then she asked me questions. Many, many questions: from my nutrition to my prenatal care, from my sleep patterns to my personal relationships, from my previous conditions to my prescription medicines.

After the last question, she put her hand on my shoulder and said, "I know how you feel."

I believed her. I knew she did.

Then she said, "First, you should know this isn't in your mind. I know there are real reasons you've been feeling so lousy, and we're going to find them."

What a relief to hear those words. I sobbed at being comforted.

At this point, she did something I had never experienced before with a doctor. She opened my chart, laid it out in front of me, and explained what my blood work showed, step by step. She then took a drop of my blood, put it on a glass slide, and projected it on a screen so I could see exactly what she was describing. She educated me about hormone levels and thyroid screenings, and pointed out that my progesterone level was very close to zero. My thyroid was also underfunctioning. She informed me that any huge imbalance of hormones could wreak havoc on the whole system, including the nervous system. She arranged for me to do a longer-term hormone test, which was done by sampling saliva over a period of twenty-eight days. The test sounded sick, but . . . so was I. She also immediately put me on natural progesterone and various herbal and vitamin supplements that supported my lymphatic system, kidneys, liver, and thyroid.

She looked at me warmly and said, "I think you're going to feel better starting tomorrow. But I should explain. This will help the physical problems. I feel there's more involved with your depression."

Depression, which can be triggered by a hormonal imbalance, often brings up emotional issues that need to be dealt with on a separate level. She suggested that the hormone replacement she was prescribing would make me feel better physically and that I could take antidepressants to stabilize my emotions. But she cautioned me that I probably would not recover fully unless I faced my emotional issues, which had surfaced through the hormone imbalance. I had already suspected this, but now she was confirming that I needed to recover in all ways.

Before I left the office that day I was weepy again, but this time it was not from sorrow. I was a woman who had just received a "not guilty" verdict from the jury on depression. I wasn't an inadequate mother and the depression wasn't caused by me. I wasn't weak, or selfish, or coldhearted. I felt I had found a doctor who listened in all ways: with her ears, her intellect, and her heart. I felt nurtured and supported. I was going to get some help and nothing, for the first time, seemed more important to me. I knew that eventually everything I cherished—my marriage, my children, my relationships, my businesses, my charity work—would be compromised unless I took the time to fix myself first. The best part was, I didn't have to figure it out on my own.

◆

There's a well-known story about a small girl who wanted a bike. Her father encouraged her to save all her coins to buy it. She did extra household chores and saved all the change she earned in a glass jar. The father, seeing her honest effort, felt great compassion and took her to the store to pick out a bike. Sitting on the seat of the exact bicycle she wanted, the little girl burst into tears. When her father asked why, she told him she'd saved much less than the bike cost. Then the father told the child to give him all the money she had saved, along with a hug, and he would pay for the rest of the bike.

Leaving Judith's office that afternoon, I thought about this story. I know it's a metaphor for God's assistance in our honest efforts to help ourselves. I can only guess how much longer I would have struggled on alone before I felt any improvement whatsoever. But Judith Moore saw my desire for answers and my willingness to tell the truth about what was really going on. Through her knowledge and understanding, she, in effect, bought the rest of the bike for me. But it's one thing to have a bike, and another thing to ride it. I knew it would take focus on my part to get better. I would have to find a new balance, push the pedals myself, and steer into the future. I knew there would be spills ahead, but I was at least moving forward.

18

◆

Is That My Inner Voice, or Did I Swallow My Cell Phone?

My daughter Brianna was still a baby herself, not even two, when Matthew was born, yet she claimed him as her baby, or her "Bubby," even before his arrival. When he was just starting to crawl, I would have to keep an eye on her, because she believed she was so much bigger than Matthew that she could pick him up and carry him. In truth, he was such a solid little guy that by age five months he weighed only a couple of pounds less than Brianna. To her great frustration, every time she tried to hold him in her arms he always managed to squirm away.

One afternoon, after I had given Matthew a bottle and he had fallen asleep, I told Brianna if she sat on the couch she could hold him on her lap. I laid the baby across her little legs, stacked pillows around them both, and started working on something else. I didn't think it would last for more than two minutes, but she sat there, completely content, patting his belly, talking to him, and kissing his head. Finally, after thirty minutes the baby woke up and I went to get him.

When Brianna got down off the couch to follow me into the kitchen, she slid right to the floor. She looked startled for a moment and then with a whimper pointed to her legs and said, "My legs are ow-ie."

Her legs had fallen completely to sleep under the weight of her baby brother. It seemed that Brianna's maternal instinct and need to nurture was stronger than her survival instinct, just like her mother's. The maternal instinct can be so all consuming that we in essence allow other parts of ourselves to fall asleep under its influence: our intellect, our social needs, our passions, and even our health. Once deadened for any length of time, these parts of our lives can be forgotten. To bring life back to our numbed existences means living with discomfort as the circulation returns.

I felt a physical improvement rather quickly following my appointment with Dr. Moore. The hormone replacement and supplements she had advised me to take seemed to be restoring balance to my system. One of the supplements she suggested for me was a green powder that you mix into a glass of water and drink. The powder is made of sprouted grains, dried vegetables, and herbs, which help to purify the liver and kidneys. The benefits proved to be excellent. You know how people ask, Why is it that everything bad for you tastes so good? All I can say is this drink must be really, really good for you. It tastes like a horse stable smells, and it looks like the water in the bottom of a flower vase after it has sat in a sunny window for two weeks. Does that tell you how desperate I was to get better?

One morning at the studio, during a daily briefing in my dressing room, the producers, writers, and Donny started making comments about the green drink I was sipping. Some mooed, others did horse whinnies, and I think a verse of "Old MacDonald" was sung. As payback, I decided to mix a green drink for everybody at the table. That's right. My name was Misery, and I wanted some company. I was very enthusiastic as I heaped the green powder into everyone's drinking water and said, "Hey, this is really healthy. I'd like to share it." Most of them just took one sip to be polite, grimaced, and didn't touch it again. Donny, never one to turn down a dare from me (it's an Osmond thing), took a huge gulp, acted like it was fine for about two seconds, then had a dramatic gag-reflex reaction. His eyes started watering, and he had to run out of the room. Only three of us tried to drink it down. We found that taking a small sip then eating four or five M&Ms to cut the taste was most effective. It probably also cut the benefits. I've heard the expression "It's a bitter pill to swallow" many times before. With the increasing popularity of these types of natural remedies, it's now "a bitter twenty ounces to swallow." Let me tell you, this nutritional drink put the "hell" in "healthy." Almost everything else Dr. Moore prescribed for me came in capsule form, for which I was thankful.

Besides the hormonal, vitamin, and herbal supplements she gave me, she also encouraged me to pay closer attention to my nutrition, get more physical exercise, and catch a couple more hours of sleep when I could. She took a look at all the choices I was making that may have played a part in my postpartum depression. She made me aware that the very foods that I was grabbing for quick energy—carbohydrates, sugars, and processed foods—were actually depleting my stamina. My chocolate cravings were constant, but satisfying the craving actually had a negative effect. It's difficult for a healthy body to process this type of diet, so for a woman who is suffering from depression it is especially exhausting. Judith explained to me that processed foods, foods that the human system doesn't recognize because they aren't natural, block the absorption of nutrients that help balance the hormonal system and the nervous system. I have come to understand how awareness of nutritional balance and attention to diet are crucial in helping to maintain emotional as well as physical health. I believe that many of the food products in our grocery stores are so chemically engineered or genetically altered that the possibility of getting enough nutrients is becoming more remote. I learned that though I was eating plenty of food, I was actually malnourished from lack of natural nutrients that my body could absorb. Even my allergic reaction to wheat was not really to the whole grain but the processed form in which I was consuming it. (Dr. Judith has included a complete description of the diet she recommended for me, along with details on the effects of nutritional choices on the postpartum body, at the end of this book.)

Not only did I begin to question how my diet was compromising my health, I also looked closely at what my children were eating and the consequences of their diet on everything from moodiness to hyperactivity. I was still in a place where shopping and preparing meals were beyond what I could do. What I was able to do early on was make better choices about foods I made available to myself and my children. It's as easy to peel open a banana as it is to open a bag of chocolate chip cookies. It may not be as much fun in the moment, but neither are the sugar crashes and raging headaches that can result when your body is screaming out for something it can use. (Although coming off sugar can be rough.)

◆

Within a week of my visit to Dr. Judith, many of the people who worked closely with me noted my improvement. The shaking feeling I had endured for months, along with the unpredictable emotions that had invaded my days, began to let up, and my ability to concentrate improved greatly. My anxiety level decreased, and my heart was no longer racing.

Though its rate may have slowed, my heart still had an undeniable, deep ache. The overpowering physical imbalances that had thrown me into PPD were on the mend, but I found myself still in a dark void emotionally. I had become aware of too much to remain emotionally asleep, oblivious to the burdens that had caused my inner self to go numb. I couldn't shut out the voice of the desperate girl I had tried to abandon in the coastal motel room. I arrived at this difficult conclusion during a celebration of my life.

For my fortieth birthday, Brian planned a surprise party at a local comedy club in Utah and invited my business associates and many friends whom I hadn't seen since moving to L.A. I thought we were going out to eat with LuAnn and Mike Samuelian, which is what I said I really wanted to do for my birthday, just a low-key celebration with our dear neighbors. When we walked into the club, over one hundred people were there to cheer me over the hill. I was really taken by surprise. As much as I loved everyone who had come to the party, my initial impulse was to turn and run. I knew that as supportive as they all were, they would also be full of concern and questions about what I was going through. Since I felt I was still struggling on a day-to-day basis, I was not ready to respond to their concern. At the same time, their evident care for me was reassuring. I felt pressured to reassure them in return that I was back to being me, full of carefree exuberance. But I couldn't. I was far from being back to the Marie they knew, and I couldn't pretend otherwise with these people. I might have been able to convince one of my friends that everything was okay, but there wasn't a chance I could do the same for all. I was present, but it was like being half in and half out of my body. They would see through it eventually. That's why I wanted to run.

Brian had planned a slide presentation of my first forty years, which was a touching gesture, but I felt uneasy having so much attention paid to my life history. I imagined a whole scenario in which by age seven people would be dozing off, by age twenty-eight the room would be half empty, and by age forty they would be rolling out the dead bodies. That didn't happen; they all stayed through to the last slide. I guess my friends have a pain tolerance that is equal to mine.

The evening was full of many laughs from personal stories. I remember listening to them and watching the slides, each representing a part of my life: a photo of the entertainer Marie, a story of the mother Marie, the doll designer Marie, the daughter, the sister, the business partner. It seemed I had played each of those roles successfully. I had memorized them well. My life was full to the brim already, but I had to ask myself, What would my life be if I didn't have a role to play? How could I describe myself outside of these roles? What defined me as an individual? I had gone from a little girl who was her mother's helper to a businesswoman who took care of her coworkers, to a wife who took care of her husband, to a mother who took care of her children. That evening made it clear to me that I needed to move on to another level. I had to become a woman who took care of herself. With Dr. Judith's help, I was taking care of my physical imbalance, but my emotions were still in chaos. I may have thought I had shut the door on those unanswered questions from the little girl inside of me. I had tried to leave her in the motel room on the California coast, but she was still inside, wanting attention, and would be alive as long as I was. It was time to seek more help.

◆

A number of years ago, after I finished a Broadway run playing Maria in *The Sound of Music*, I went through a brief period of time when I was unable to sing without crying. When I started a song, my throat would become choked with emotion. I even was forced to cancel an upcoming concert appearance. Singing is a vulnerable thing to do. There isn't any other human expression exactly like it. It's creating music, and music must have feeling behind it to be effective. I think a person can only bury their true feelings for so long before they make their presence known one way or another. When this was happening in my life, I was connected with a reputable family counselor who practiced near my hometown in Utah. She had helped me process my emotions and deal with the effect they were having on my singing career. I decided to call her again.

At the end of the first session, which was a very long phone call from L.A., she said to me, "Marie, you are so masterful at perceiving and filling the needs of others. You can't do that anymore, because your needs aren't being met." She suggested to me that depression, even PPD, is friendly if we pay attention to it. It's a way for our subconscious to inform our conscious that our lives are out of whack and that there are things that need changing. Countless women, she explained, suffer depression that stems from suppressing their feelings, yet the odd thing is, some don't even know they're doing it or that they're depressed. They just think that life has to be that way. I know that I had accepted it for myself with a "that's life" attitude for a long time.

The most eye-opening moment came for me when she related that the women she had worked with over the years who suffered from PPD had a noticeable common factor. Many had been victims of emotional abuse or suffered sexual abuse as children. Women with this history tend to deal with it by attempting to control their lives in every aspect. She explained that it's the reason I loved to work. I could understand that in my life. I felt the most relaxed in a very disciplined atmosphere. She told me that the hormonal imbalances following birth, as well as the unpredictable nature of taking care of a new baby, cause these women to feel out of control. These factors alone can cause depression in a person with no history of abuse. So it can quickly bring deeper issues to the surface for the woman who had been abused. I saw that this had happened to me as well. The hormonal imbalance following my baby's birth had shifted my body chemistry, which caused my emotions to be unpredictable. Once my emotions were out of balance, I felt I no longer had the means to suppress all the hurt and pain that I had hidden away for years. And then I was left with no option except to clean up everything that had spilled out of my inner self. It seems PPD didn't just appear out of nowhere, and it wouldn't disappear into nowhere. As painful or as far in my past as the abuse was, I would not be able to fully heal until I acknowledged those experiences for what they were. I had to look at them for myself and put them in proper context, not as shameful, but as unjustified abuse.

This was the last thing I wanted to do. I had been through it once. Did I have to relive the pain? I had hoped the solution would be simpler.

That's not what I was hearing. She was telling me in the most forthright way possible that healing from a depression doesn't happen with a wish. It takes a willingness to look at your problems and relentless determination to go through the pain of self-examination, to uncover the dis-ease that is causing the depression. Most of all it takes time. Lots of it. She proposed that I start to change how I felt about myself by acknowledging the child inside of me, the inner voice that I had suppressed so long ago, and listening to her again.

I think for women who are mothers, the idea of giving any time to yourself is very hard to grasp. I made a sideways observation about my lack of personal time during one of the *Donny & Marie* shows. We were talking about *Sesame Street* characters and choosing the one we most identified

with. I remarked that I would be Oscar the Grouch, because
the only time I have five minutes to myself is when I'm in
the can. After that show aired, I received a handful of e-mails
from mothers with little ones at home asking, "Hey, how do
you even manage that? My toddler follows me right into the
bathroom."

The to-do list I have at home could probably wrap
around the house twice. I know this is true for most of my
friends too. As soon as one thing is checked off, another appears. Like gray hair . . . pull one and four take its place.

So when you tell a woman to take time for herself, her response is most likely going to be, "When?" That's how I felt.
If I was lucky enough to set aside thirty minutes to myself,
just then one of the kids would take a tumble off a bike and
need to have a skinned knee cleaned and bandaged. Almost
like the unproven law of rain: If you carry an umbrella all
day, not a drop will fall. But if there isn't a cloud in the sky
and you venture out without one, that's when you'll be
caught in a spontaneous downpour with a flash flood that
rips the suede right off your favorite pair of shoes.

Pharmaceutical companies have wised up to the constant
pressure most women are under. They have recognized
mothers as a captive audience of consumers and started running commercials for antidepressants on television. "Are you
stressed and anxious, worried and exhausted?" the commercials ask. May I just say for all women: "Duh!!!" Like the
commercials for Compoz from my mother's era, these ads
make medication sound like a quick fix. Who doesn't want
pain to disappear quickly?

The idea of taking a pill to make depression go away is
very appealing, but it sidesteps the cause and treats only the
symptoms, like a bandage that only hides an infection. Unless we can acknowledge the feelings we are covering up, it
will only be a matter of time before the depression returns in

a different form. It's not that I'm against antidepressants. In some cases a person may need them to produce neuro-transmitters in the same way a diabetic needs insulin. They can be used to treat a lifelong physiological problem. In other cases, I think they can help to settle the mind down, calm the rough waves of our emotions, and provide a plat-form from which a person can work on what she needs to do to make changes in how she functions. It was tempting to just take something to numb the emotional pain so I could get through my days. But for me, the thought of having se-vere depression return was worse than taking the time to work out my underlying feelings now.

◆

I decided to start mothering myself in whatever small ways I could. I was going to pay attention to my needs by giving my inner voice a chance to be heard. Changing a lifelong pat-tern is difficult, but I knew I couldn't continue down the same path I had been on. I had to acknowledge my feelings. That wasn't going to be any walk in the park, but I had to get off the emotional merry-go-round, going up and down with-out gaining any self-awareness. As a child, I loved the scene in the Julie Andrews–Dick Van Dyke movie *Mary Poppins* in which the horses leave the carousel and bounce across the rolling hills, carrying their riders to new terrain. But in real life, new terrain can be frightening and cause a lot of confu-sion because you have to leave the circular path you have traveled for so long.

The first leap I took outside of the circle was to state my own needs out loud, to myself. Then, once I had done that, I followed up with a way I could take care of that need. For ex-ample, one afternoon between taping the first and second *Donny & Marie* shows, I began feeling deeply pensive and could sense that darkness closing in on me again. I knew I was exhausted from the start. I had been up almost the whole night before because one of my kids had an upset stomach. I was late getting into the studio, and as soon as I walked in I had about five large business issues to deal with, scheduling conflicts, and calls that needed responses. My "mommy" phone rang continuously. I got a call from my daughter that her cheerleading sneaker had fallen apart during practice and could someone bring her another pair? My son remembered that he needed a pinewood derby car made for Cub Scouts . . . tomorrow! My two-year-old had to tell me she was wearing big-girl panties today. To me, these were the important calls.

I made it through the first show before it all started to unravel for me. So I closed my dressing-room door for a minute and said out loud to myself: "I know you're tired and your back is aching. You've been up all night and you've had to deal with problems since sunrise. I know that you feel bad. But please. I need a little more from you. I have to get through the second show. I promise that tonight, after the kids go to bed, I'll light some aromatherapy candles and you can soak for at least twenty minutes in a hot mineral-salt bath. I'll take care of you."

I admit it was a bit odd at the beginning to speak out loud to myself. If I was at work, I would step into the bathroom, turn on the exhaust fan, and hope no one would think I had lost it altogether. At least in the car I could pretend I was singing along to the radio. Let me tell you, once I cut the voice of that inner child loose, she wanted to gab day and night. But it was necessary at first to be sure I was listening to my own needs and giving my feelings validity. I can honestly say that this method started to work for me. I found that I felt better as soon as I acknowledged my feelings instead of pushing them to the side. However, following up on what I promised myself was often the most challenging part, because it involved time . . . of which I had exactly . . . none.

For me to do something nurturing for myself meant that someone else was going to have to sacrifice whatever I would have been doing for them during that time. It would require saying the word *no* once in a while, which is still hard for me to do.

It sounds harmless enough to say, "No, I can't. I promised myself a hot bath tonight." But I'm a person who finds it difficult to relax or even work if I know someone I love is upset or unhappy. I had to make myself follow through when I said no in the same way a parent disciplines a child. If you say no to a child and then reverse your decision and give in, she will always expect you to give in, or pester you until you do. The same was true of saying yes to myself. Even if it was uncomfortable, I had to respect my own needs. How could I expect my children, my husband, or my coworkers and friends to respect what I needed to do for myself if I didn't?

When I expressed these thoughts to my counselor, she told me that probably millions of women felt very similar about their self-worth. One of the topics she brought up was authority. "Women," she said, "tend to believe that authority is outside of themselves. They feel that someone other than them has the right answer, or knows better than they do."

Looking back, the fourth day after my baby was born I truly knew that I wasn't just experiencing the baby blues, but I downplayed my own instinctual feelings, assumed my doctor was the authority, and followed his instructions. Not to place fault, because a doctor can only know how to help if you give him or her full information. But I didn't trust that what I was feeling was worthy of mentioning. I didn't give myself enough credit to believe what my gut was telling me. (And without a doubt, it was a much bigger gut than before

I was pregnant.) I was so afraid of not being heard and not having what I was going through validated that I went almost six months before I sought more help. Dr. Moore was a breath of fresh air for me because she encouraged me to have the authority to acknowledge what I was experiencing. She never negated my feelings. Instead, she would use them as a place to start diagnosing, which gave me the courage to tell her the truth.

I knew I had to find a way to be grounded in my own authority. I could no longer use being a mother, or working, or even someone else's opinion to escape the complexities of my real needs. I already trusted my maternal instincts and my business instincts; now I had to learn to trust my intuition about myself. It had fallen asleep under the weight of my pressing it down. Once I took away the restraint, my intuitive feelings started coming back to life. It was indeed uncomfortable and even painful as the circulation came back into my sleeping soul. Sometimes the healing process felt almost bigger than me, like my little Brianna trying to pick up the baby. My issues were both heavy and almost impossibly stubborn. However, as much as I squirmed to get away from being elevated to a higher consciousness, it held on to me, patting my swallowed shame and kissing my defeated head until I agreed to wake up to what my life could be.

19

◆

Christmas Mourning

Christmas. Christmas. Christmas. I love it. I love every sentimental, generous, surprising, decadent, tree-trimming, overeating minute of it. I love to hunt for great gifts, I love to surprise people, and did I mention I love food? So Christmas is my holiday of heaven. I am capital *O* overenthusiastic about Christmas.

When my first two kids, Stephen and Jessica, were still little, I found a needlepoint pattern for Christmas stockings that I thought was adorable. It was an old-fashioned Christmas scene with a tree loaded up with gifts and a little girl or boy looking out of a window to see Santa in his sleigh. Across the top of the stocking is room for the child's name to be spelled out. It was a delicate and time-consuming project; each stocking took countless hours. I carried them with me all year long and would pull them out during any spare moment I had just to finish the first two. When my third baby, Rachael, came along, I knew that I couldn't leave her out. She had to have an identical stocking too. I'm sure you can see the outcome of this story, four additional kids later. I have since regretted my decision to needlepoint stockings that are the size of small sleeping bags. My friends predicted that by the time I made it to stocking number seven I was going to hate the old-fashioned Christmas scene that had originally delighted me. This year I'm starting on a stocking for child number five, Brandon. Brianna and Matthew may not get theirs until they graduate from high school. After the fourth one I was thinking, "Why did I have to pick seven-letter names for all of my children? By the time I was finishing the *L* in Michael's name, I wondered how I would explain my carpal tunnel to the doctor: "No, not a computer. Would you believe a stocking? . . . and I don't mean from pulling pantyhose on every day." In desperation I might change the names of my last three kids to Sy, Jo, and Al. Or maybe I'll keep their names and change to iron-on letters.

But I press on toward my goal: a photo of all seven children, each holding a personalized, Mom-made stocking on Christmas morning. I don't care if Stephen is twenty-nine years old with a family of his own by the time I get them all done. He will come home and pose in his pajamas with all the other kids!

Christmas, the season of sensory overload, is not the best time for working on taking care of your own life in any manner. Sticking to a healthy diet when you're surrounded by sugar in every possible form and finding personal time between parties sounds good, but these are about as possible for me as adding a handwritten note to every Christmas card, which I also dream of doing.

We taped shows until the Friday before Christmas, which gave me little time to prepare for the holiday. We wanted to spend Christmas in Utah, near the rest of our families, but wouldn't be able to get there until just days before. I was quickly starting to feel overwhelmed. I had to put thought into gifts for not only my family, but all of my professional associates as well, and I was feeling very little Christmas spirit. I was still operating in a world where just doing the shows, taking care of the children, and trying to stay on the program Dr. Judith had suggested was all I could do . . . and I had days when that fell apart.

One morning I got the older kids out the door to school and I was changing and feeding the little ones when I started to feel kind of fuzzy, like after a big Sunday meal when you want to take a long nap kind of fuzzy. I felt really relaxed. In fact, way too relaxed for a woman who needed to be at the studio in less than an hour. I was drop-dead tired, to be precise. I realized what had happened before I even looked in my medicine case. In my rush, I had grabbed a sleep aid Dr. Judith had given me to take on the nights when my racing mind wouldn't let me rest. I had taken one of those instead of the thyroid supplement that I took every morning. Let's just say it was much safer for Brian to drive me into the studio, and I think I even slept through having my makeup put on. I tried an ice pack, eyedrops, even an exorbitant amount of chocolate to get me pepped up. It was one of the most enjoyable and easy shows I've ever done. I was so laid-back that everything moved along effortlessly. Donny thought it was especially great. It was the first time I laughed at every one of his jokes.

After taping the last two shows that week and distributing and exchanging gifts at work, I was depleted of all my spare energy. I still had to shop for family and close friends, and the people in my office in Utah. I knew by the time we packed up the kids and got to Utah, I would have less than a week to prepare for Christmas. I wanted to go home and crawl between the covers. I would have been happy to let Christmas pass me by and not get out of bed again until the new millennium, and I'm talking about the year 3000! Here

I was, trying to come to grips with what I needed to do to get myself through PPD, and I was being plunged into the season of high expectations.

The rigorous schedule and the discipline it took to pull it all off completely sapped the spontaneity and the joy right out of the season for me. I never had to "try" to be happy during the holidays before, but this year was a monumental effort in every way. As we packed up the car in L.A. and started the drive to Utah, I sensed that I had shifted my feelings again into a remote place. I didn't have the time or even the patience to listen to my own heart. I felt like I had the expectations of my babies resting on my shoulders to make Christmas as special as it always had been. It began to feel like a maddening circle. I was already experiencing waves of guilt that my family and friends were going to be disappointed, and the sadness that came with the guilt left me feeling alienated from any spirit of celebration.

One of the most nurturing gifts I received Christmas week was provided by my associates. Knowing that my schedule was tight, Lisa, my creative director and doll partner, and my insightful neighbor Linda, who had rescued me after the baby shower, had taken action to make sure I didn't come home to a Christmas-less house.

Everyone at the Utah office had purchased a gorgeous Christmas tree, complete with decorations, and arranged to have my good friend John Walker put it up in my living room. Linda, in her magnificent way, had put her loving touch into decorating the inside of the house from top to bottom. Being able to cross that off my list gave me the boost I needed to finish other Christmas preparations.

I can't say if it was having time away from work or being around all of my extended family and the memories that I share with them, but I was bombarded by more unpredictable emotions, mostly feelings of deep sorrow, which came in the midst of the celebrating. My resistance to the downward spiral was weakening again. It was as if I were mourning a passing. It was the passing of the Marie who allowed her true voice to be squashed. She had spent thirty-seven years in exile from her own thoughts and feelings, and now that was over, and I couldn't even pretend she still existed. The mourning was apparently going to happen right then, without any consideration for it being Christmas.

PPD was changing me profoundly. It was opening me up to take an in-depth look at every area of my life: my careers, the *Donny & Marie* show, living in Los Angeles, my work relationships, and the people I surrounded myself with—every one of them. I questioned why I wanted to perform, why I wanted to have my other businesses, and the choices I had made residing in Los Angeles, from the community I lived in to whom I was allowing in my house. I questioned my own motives for keeping unhealthy relationships in my life. I had to ask myself why I had allowed my feelings to be trampled on by certain coworkers, neighbors, and even friends and relatives. I thought for hours about the power of money, to either hurt or help. I reevaluated all of my priorities. Were they in the order that I wanted them in?

I considered my faith in God. I searched my heart as to whether I was still living according to His purpose for my life or denying His creation by allowing myself to exist in a half life.

I devoted much thought to my relationship with my brothers and my parents. Did we know and appreciate one another as adults? Or had we grown up working together but not really communicating? Could we now let history be just that and see ourselves as individuals with a deep blood bond that had proven to be undeniable?

I took a magnified look at each of my children. I've always thought of motherhood as a partnership with God, and believed that He has entrusted me with their care. Were they secure? Did they have worries? Were they getting the attention they needed individually? Because of my work schedule, had I convinced myself at their expense that it was all about "quality" time when what they really craved was "quantity" time? Was the postpartum depression going to have a longer-lasting impact on their lives than on my own?

I looked at my relationship with Brian. I opened my eyes to all the issues that we had pushed away as inconsequential. Once I looked, I found them all, still there, submerged in a sea of hurt feelings and anger. It's public knowledge that Brian and I went through a separation shortly after that Christmas that lasted for six months. I've heard the gamut of opinions about our choice to separate, just as I've heard opinions on all the other choices I've made in my life. I've had people tell me I didn't really have postpartum depression but that I was in a bad marriage. I've heard that Brian felt neglected and that my work took over our lives. The tabloids blamed everything from my doll business to Mel Gibson to a lemon-water diet from my teenage years.

The real reason was not that black and white. It was both simpler and more complicated than any one reason. You aren't in a marriage for thirteen years and allow any one thing to cause discord. It was never a question of devotion for each other, it was more about looking at our individual changes in those thirteen years and realizing that we had postponed one too many times the basis of a healthy relationship—true communication. We had shut down and started living separate but parallel lives. We couldn't see what the other even needed or was about because there were miles between our paths. Unhappiness is not an overnight occurrence in a marriage; it's a buildup of denied feelings and stale routines and habits that no longer serve their original purpose.

In the same way that I described to my children the image of individual health as represented by the four legs of a chair, I think of marriage as two pillars, equally strong and both supporting the same house. You can't let one lean or topple without risking the structure of the whole house. The pillars weather storms together because there is a unique balance between them that gives strength to the house. I feel that marriage consists of two people being one in purpose, one in mind, and one in heart.

Our marriage had been compromised by a number of things, and probably at the top of the list was my inability to express my true needs. Brian conveyed to me recently that he felt ineffectual in being able to help me. He told me, "When you cried and cried and wouldn't tell me what was wrong, I was left with my hands tied." After a while a man just stops asking what's needed, and begins to bury and store hurt feelings.

The separation was necessary. I was angry and Brian was miserable. We needed the time apart, without communication early on, to focus on ourselves and the individual parts we had played in our marriage troubles instead of continuing to be critical of each other. With introspection came personal discovery about what our priorities were and what we had allowed them to be replaced with over time. Brian did a lot of internal work on his own; at the same time I continued my own reflection on what my future held. We did set a date and time to see each other again because I believe that too much time apart leads to building more walls around the hurt and pain that you may not be able to see over as time passes. I knew that we couldn't truly work things out between us if we weren't together to do it.

When we saw each other again, we came to the table with humility and softened hearts. I was able to see Brian's love for me and his undying devotion to our children. I still had fears about renewing the relationship. But little by little we let the walls down and chipped away at the awful fear that it would be only a matter of time before we fell into the patterns that had given us reason to separate.

Perhaps our saving grace in all of this was that we truly loved our children and were equally committed to each other and to working at repairing our injured relationship.

The details are a matter of privacy, and we have to honor and protect our personal lives, but we have learned the most important skill in marriage: communication. Honest communication dispels fear, and once fear is gone, true intimacy can occur. I do know from experience that with effort, open-mindedness, and a lot of prayer, people can change, hearts can heal, and it's possible to fall in love all over again.

A wise person once told me this about difficulty: "Live through it. Learn from it. Move on." It's really the only positive choice we have.

20

Pull Up a Chair

My baby is walking away from me. Less than a week after Matthew's first birthday, he pulled himself into a standing position using the edge of my chair and turned to look at his goal. Brian would like to think he was the goal, but I'm pretty sure it was the cookie he happened to be holding. As Matthew stepped off, his arms waved out to the sides, unsure of how they could be helpful this far from the floor. His diapered bottom swayed side to side, making his balance unstable with each step. He made it about four full steps before he plunged forward into his father's arms; his eyes lit up with excitement.

Now he's all over the place. Up and down the stairs, exploring from room to room, having no concept of his limitations. If I let him, I'm sure he would follow the older kids right out the front door for school, with a look on his face as if to say, "Hey, where's my backpack?" (Or, as each of my kids called it during their preschool years "my pa-pack.")

I watch my other little ones, Brandon and Brianna, experience their lives. Their natural tendency, ungoverned, is to explore and learn through experience. Everything in their path has equal potential for their fascinated examination, from the simplest knob on a dresser drawer to the stones lining a walkway. They have to touch, move, smell, taste, hold, turn, push, or pull any object that catches their attention.

Recently, while we were packing the car to drive from Los Angeles to Utah, Brianna discovered the full range of her power. I was checking what the other kids were packing when I heard the garage door going up and down. I assumed it was Brian putting the bikes and yard toys in the garage until I realized the door had gone up and down at least four times. I went to the front door to see what on earth was going on. Brianna was standing on the front seat of my car, remote in hand, with a look on her face as if she had just figured out how to launch the space shuttle.

I am rediscovering the joy of being alive now, in this moment, in this hour, and in this day through my children, especially my three youngest. Small children can capture the attention of a room full of adults, I think because they show us the pure happiness of a simple accomplishment, the unself-conscious laughter in a funny moment, and how to live without fear. They are innocent in their intentions and untouched by the reality of life experience. As we get older it seems we lose faith in our ability to express ourselves as purely. Little children have a way of reminding us of our original purpose: joy.

I knew when I chose the name Matthew for my baby that its meaning was "gift of God." What I didn't know was that this tiny baby would give me the great gift of finding my true self, first through PPD, then through love, and now, ultimately, through joy.

My journey through PPD allowed me to perceive the emotion that had dominated much of my life: fear. I lived for many years afraid that who I was on the inside would never be enough. I had always felt the need to please, to fit in, to succeed, so I set aside my need and desire to explore on my own, fearing that I would fall short, make an irreversible mistake, or embarrass myself and my family. I experienced pain, as we all do, each time I felt rejection. But then, because of these fears, I made it worse by rejecting myself. I built a wall around the unacceptable little girl inside of me to hide her from others. Then, if that wall wasn't high enough and I didn't feel I was living up to what I thought was expected of me, I built another wall in front of the first, keeping any part of my inner self from escaping. Every time I put up a new wall, I would tell myself, more negative thoughts like, "You're no good. Stay away." Many walls later I had safely entombed the little girl so I could successfully become the person I was most comfortable being: the one who takes care of everyone, the one who can handle anything she's given. I liked the qualities of that person; I still do. The problem was I acquired them at the expense of myself. They came from fear and the need to control, not from love and the need for joy. This brought me a deep sorrow and yet was a healing teacher in my PPD experiences. I had to accept that I had treated myself in a way I would never treat anyone I loved. Could I imagine saying to my children any of the things I had told myself for years and years? Could I possibly say to my beautiful, bold, and intuitive thirteen-year-old daughter, Jessica: "You need to be more or you'll never be worthy of anyone's love." When my funny and insightful eleven-year-old, Rachael, tells me her observations on life, would I even think of saying, "Keep your thoughts to yourself. Don't you know your opinions don't count?" Could I ever tell my charming, sensitive, artistic nine-year-old son, Michael: "That drawing just isn't good enough. You can't do anything right."? It would break my heart if any of my kids thought of themselves as stupid, incapable, or unattractive. I couldn't stand to hear it, because I see each of them as the most marvelous, gifted, and stunning individual to ever exist. I would go to any extreme to keep them from negative thoughts that diminish their self-worth.

So it was a searing and painful truth to realize that I didn't put any effort into sparing myself or the little girl that huddled inside of me, knees tucked up to her chin, crying, hidden in a fortress of inaccessible walls. I had never given her a chance to be enough. She lost out on my affection before she had any chance to know her true purpose or what she had to offer.

I couldn't see to what extent I had relinquished myself to fear until my life as I knew it was shaken by PPD to the very foundation and the walls cracked wide open. What saved me from crumbling completely was my belief that the only sure foundation in my life is my faith in God. I know I wouldn't have been able to overcome and heal from PPD without prayer and the comfort and direction that comes from above. PPD was much larger than my human capabilities. I was flattened on the floor and I was not going to be able to get up until I looked at the basic elements of my life. I had to go back to the principle I try to teach my children. I had to rebuild the four legs of my chair, one by one: physical, social, mental, and spiritual.

I had to first admit that I was not physically well. My system was severely imbalanced: hormonally, chemically, nutritionally, and even environmentally, meaning I had polluted my body with years of self-abusive dieting, sleep deprivation, and physical exertion. I had to accept that I was unable to fix this on my own. I had to seek help, and this meant revealing to others that I was having problems. I made the connection with Dr. Judith Moore, who assisted me in repairing my physical self. In addition to her treatment I went for lymphatic massages and chiropractic adjustments, which aided my physical healing. Then I was able to focus on the other areas of my life.

This led me to rebuild the second leg of my chair: social interaction. I needed support from my family and friends. I allowed those I love most to know how I was feeling. I listened to the reassuring words of my mother. I let my friends help me get through the bad days. Sometimes I asked for help, but I was often graced by the gentle and loving thoughtfulness of people who lent support without any expectations and, even more incredibly, without judgment. My fears started to melt as the connection that came from sharing my experience radiated sincere love and concern back to me, and then from me out to others. I've had friends tell me that being a part of my PPD experience helped them to grow in understanding and awareness. I can honestly say, if tough times make you stronger, then I know it has applied to the bonds I have with those I love.

Once I felt that I had established a way to start physically healing and had a social support system in place, I was able to take a look at the third leg: my mental state of being. The negative thoughts I had and the severity of the emotions I was feeling were far less overwhelming once the physical problems were in check. I was also encouraged through my social contacts, my doctors, my family, and my friends—to take care of myself completely, and this meant my mental health as well. I knew it would be necessary to face issues, give voice to my fears, and confront the things I had suppressed for years. The best way for me to do this was through counseling and emotional work. Just talking about it openly brought about change for the better. I found it to be a safe place where I could honestly express my feelings, even the most tumultuous feelings brought on by PPD. Talking about my past abuses, being treated as a product and not a person, and even my anger with my husband gave room for my feelings to be acknowledged, carefully thought about, and put into perspective in my current life. I credit my PPD experience with healing my marriage, because now Brian and I are more than just surviving together. We are committed to each other and to helping each other find happiness. We have renewed our promise to communicate truthfully. The problems that arise now are discussed with love, not ignored, hidden, or controlled in fear. Nothing of lasting value comes easily, but in the end the effort is definitely worth it.

The fourth leg of the chair is the most important to me: spiritual. I know this is the one that maintains the balance of the other three. The strength of this leg is compromised only by fear, because it was built for love. I knew I couldn't heal until I gave over to God the fear that had occupied me for much of my lifetime. My PPD experience gave me the opportunity to fix the misperceptions that had caused me to conceal a part of myself inside during the first half of my life, so I wouldn't spend the second half of my life in fear. This experience helped me accept that I had tried to do everything I could to control my world, and it reminded me daily what a futile effort that was. I started to knock down my walls of fear, I found that everything I had tried so hard to suppress or deny was manageable, and that it diminished when I handled it with love. I had to look closely at each issue, see it truthfully for what it was, and decide how to deal with it. Would I let it remain, harboring resentment and self-blame, or with faith give it over to God to be healed and then released? Only then was I to establish my true boundaries. I didn't need walls of protection anymore. I am learning to use my intuition about establishing my own boundaries as a guide for my life. This still does not happen easily for me, but I know now how to set them.

I have begun to have love for myself through forgiveness.

I have forgiven myself for my postpartum depression. I am now forgiving myself for not trusting my intuition about my body and trying to ignore the warnings instead of taking time to pay attention. I am forgiving myself for the uncontrollable tears and the trip up the coast. I am forgiving myself for not being able to feel the happiness and joy that I wanted to express when I was around my new baby and my other children. I know that I love them unconditionally, and I am starting to be able to let go of the moments I may have missed with them and treasure the moments that are here today. I am still forgiving myself for my inability to keep up, to communicate fully, and to ask for what I need.

I had always prayed and felt the presence of God, but now I have gained the understanding that His offer of help is always there. I give my struggles over to His strength.

◆

All my effort and desire to be in control of my family life, my career, and my image changed in purpose when I found self-worth through love. All my concerns about being the perfect mother, wife, businesswoman, entertainer, and friend were put in a healthy perspective through love and forgiveness.

I now tell my children: "I may make mistakes, which I hope you can forgive me for. I will probably never be the perfect mother, but I will always have a perfect love for you."

That love means I want my children to continue to learn through experience, to truly know themselves, to be comfortable with who they are, and to live truthfully. I *don't* want to spare them hard work or effort. I *do* want to spare them from self-doubt and judging their worth on the perfection of the unblemished models in retouched magazine ads. I *don't* want to spare them growing pains on the road to accomplishment. I *do* want to spare them from the discouragement that comes from attempting to live up to other people's expectations instead of their own. I *don't* want to spare them the feeling of collapsing in bed at night, exhausted from a good day full of hard work and family life. I *do* want to spare them from the feeling of not being able to get out of bed in the morning because of debilitating depression. Most important, I do want them to understand balance: physical, social, mental, and spiritual. I want them to know and love God, and I want them to love themselves.

But there was one other child I needed to love perfectly. I gathered up the lost little girl inside of me, gave her a voice, cleaned her wounds, bandaged her long-broken spirit and reminded her that she was exactly the person I wanted to be. I'm beginning to understand her and because of that I can love her. I have started to let that love grow from the inside out. PPD made it unmistakably clear to me that I can't love others without first loving myself. True love can't be walled up and suppressed. Loving myself means taking care of myself. That doesn't mean being selfish or constantly on guard and protecting myself. What self-love does mean is I have to keep my balance by acknowledging what I need to be the best wife, mother, friend, businessperson, and even the best woman I can be. I'm not there yet. I know I'm a work in progress, but I am creating an environment that will nurture all my possibilities and dreams.

I'm learning to listen to my needs. I check in with Dr. Judith when I start to feel physically unbalanced. I let my husband take over at home when I feel it's too much. Now more than ever I look for ways to help other women who are also having a hard time. I don't wait to be asked, I just do what I intuitively know they need. It restores my faith to know that we each make a difference. It makes my heart beat stronger. I feel more alive. And I can forget past hurts by helping others heal.

I'm learning to say no. I say no to the things that I feel obligated to do out of guilt. I say no to people who criticize in a harmful way. I say no to living in the past, wishing something were different, and to feelings of regret.

I'm learning to say yes. I say yes to blowing off the laundry for another day to sit on the floor and play a game with my kids. I say yes to laughing at my own idiosyncrasies, enjoying who I am and my perspective on life. I say yes to pampering myself when I need to . . . a twenty-minute hot bath, an occasional massage, lunches out with my close girlfriends to catch up and just laugh. I say yes to my best friend, Brian, and the weekly date nights he arranges for just the two of us. Our kids act as if they think it's silly, but they never fail to remind us to go. I say yes to the changes that I am making every day in my perceptions and yes to educating myself about how to support and enhance those changes. I put everything else on hold and say yes when my child needs to be near me: held, comforted, and heard.

I'm learning to listen. I listen to the needs of my body. I allow myself to lie down and rest instead of pushing to do one more task. I listen to my mind. I give an ear to the whisper of my intuition. I allow myself time for solitude and reflection almost every day, even if that means sitting in the car in the grocery store parking lot for ten minutes. I write in my journal more, making a short list of what the day brought and the ways I am thankful, even if some days my only accomplishments seem to be things like getting my son a haircut, making the bed, and sorting the kids' socks. I listen to inspirational tapes and to positive, proactive people. Sometimes just having my mother tell me a silly joke can turn my day around. I do something to feed my brain every day, even if that only means reading one page of a book. I listen to the simple needs of my heart—things that took me half of my life to learn.

I believe. I believe God shows us His presence every day, from the way the earth orbits the sun, to the stars, to the change of seasons from birth to death. I see that He is about order, not chaos. I believe that God has the right sense of time for when we should grow in knowledge and understanding. He knows when we are ready. We only need to listen. It was the same with my baby's first steps. He took them when he was ready. I am as exhilarated by the path the rest of my life will take as Matthew was by his first walk across the room. And if I lose my balance, I will topple into the loving arms of my Father in Heaven. For now, I am up off of the floor and balanced over the four legs of a new chair. It may take me a while to get used to the change of perspective it has given me in every area of my life, but I like the way it is supporting me. I have also found that there's a bountiful common table where we can find everything we need to nourish our bodies, nurture ourselves and others, sustain our growth through learning, and strengthen our spirits. All we need to do is pull up a sturdy chair.

Epilogue Poem

This poem came to my mind in a moment of sincere prayer, and I wrote it down. Its message was forty years in the making and will now be forty years in the living.

> We strive for power, displaying strength,
> Hiding fear deep beneath.
> Finally, sorrow brings truth, too much to bear;
> In Christ we find relief.
>
> Our trials bring pain,
> Show weakness, shame;
> Too hard life's burdens seem.
> Give over fear, peace will appear,
> Then learn thy self, esteem.

Marie Osmond

Marie's List of PPD Symptoms

There were a number of very late nights we (Marcia and I) spent writing this book. Usually, around two-thirty or three A.M., any thoughts of seriousness about the task at hand would disappear as fast as an open bag of potato chips. It is in those moments, when laughter took the place of sleep, that our bizarre senses of humor would make their presence most known. I wanted to share some of the results.

Your emotions change so quickly your mood ring explodes on your finger.

At Halloween, none of the neighborhood kids want to trick-or-treat at the "scary lady's" house.

You take a Lean Cuisine out of the freezer and eat it for lunch before you remember to microwave it.

You contemplate how long it would take to drown in the lawn sprinkler.

◆

You couldn't find the energy to answer the doorbell even if the Publishers Clearing House van was parked in your driveway.

◆

The love songs that used to make you cry now make you want to shout, "Oh, give me a break!"

◆

You feel so rotten, vultures are perched on your mailbox, waiting for you.

◆

The neighborhood association informs you that your house is not zoned for the one hundred and twenty personalities living inside you.

◆

Your bathrobe permanently takes on the shape of your body.

◆

Telemarketers hang up on *you*.

◆

Your newborn liked you so much better from the inside.

◆

It's been so long since you washed your hair that the directions on your shampoo bottle have been changed to "Lather. Rinse. Repeat. Repeat. Repeat. Repeat."

◆

When your mother offers to "hold the baby," you crawl into her arms.

◆

You would be the perfect test subject for waterproof mascara.

◆

You call it a major accomplishment if you hold out forty minutes between crying jags.

◆

Your baby's first words are, "Take my mother. . . . Please!"

◆

Shirley MacLaine's got nothing on you. You're having a permanent "out-of-body" experience.

◆

Your baby's father is so afraid to come home he has supplies lowered to you from a hovering helicopter.

◆

When you finally put on a little makeup and brush your hair, your baby has no idea who you are.

BOOK SUBTITLES, CONSIDERED AND REJECTED

PPD Does Not Stand for Pretty Porcelain Dolls

If Misery Loves Company, Why Am I Here Alone?

I Think It's Just Gas

Road Rage? I Invented It

Post Partum Depression for Dummies

If Only My Bills Were As Low As My Mood

How to Lose Three Pounds of Water Weight By Crying for 24 Hours

I Shot J.R.

NY PPD Blue!

Up the PCH with PPD

Life Is Just What PPD Makes It

Kids Do the Darnedest Things to Your Body

If You Don't Like My Mood, Stick Around for Five Minutes, It'll Change

Simple Abundance, My Mosaic!

The PPD Makeover: Including Hormonal Chin Hair Styling

Pull the Estrogen Mask Firmly Toward Your Face, the Bags Under Your Eyes Will Not Inflate

The One Thing Super Glue Can't Fix

I Wasn't Running Away, I Just Missed My Exit

Hanging on Through Postpartum Depression Ruined My Manicure

Marie's PPD First Aid Kit

◆

The kit should be large enough to carry the proper contents needed in a PPD emergency yet small enough to be mobile . . . any mother's purse will do. Avoid using a diaper bag; you will get stares when your bottle of antidepressants is right next to the baby's bottle.

The contents should be arranged so that the most desired aid can be found quickly without unpacking the entire kit. This means chocolate in a bag attached to the handle, got it?

Your PPD First Aid Kit should contain the following:

- *One unit:* Snug-fitting earplugs. These are to be used when well-meaning family members and associates tell you to "snap out of it."

- *One unit:* Tissues. These should be "with lotion" to prevent nose-skin removal (unless you're one of those lucky women who can cry without your nose running).

- *One unit:* Oversized Jackie O. sunglasses. These will hide the top half of your face if you absolutely have to go out in public.

- *One unit:* Black felt bag with two eyeholes cut out. This is an emergency item, used if a friend or family member wants to take your picture with the baby. A pillowcase can be a substitute, however, the fit is not as good. *Do not drive while wearing bag.*

- *One unit:* Wire cutters. These come in handy for snipping the cord on a pesky ringing phone without having to bend over to remove it from the jack.

- *Two units:* Muumuus. For an emergency clothing dilemma. These pull easily over the head, hide almost everything, and will keep you from being arrested for public nudity.

- *One unit:* Makeup bag. This is not for makeup anymore. This is to hold all your small bottles: hormone replacements, antidepressants, ibuprofen, eyedrops, oh . . . and one lipstick. (Remember what my mother said: "No matter what, wear lipstick!") The lipstick can also be used to write "go away" on your bedroom door.

- *One unit:* Baby-sized pillow. This is not for your baby. Place your own face in the pillow if you feel a scream coming on. The pillow will muffle the noise and prevent concern from your neighbors.

- *One unit:* Bag of chips, pretzels, or cheese curls. This is to go with the above-mentioned chocolate for salt/sugar-craving emergencies.

- *One unit:* A photo of you from high school, college, wedding day, any pre-baby photo will do. This is to remind you that you did have a brain and a personality at one time.

ADDITIONAL TIPS:

1. Do not apply direct pressure to your injured sense of self, you have enough outside pressure.
2. Protect your wounded heart from the poisonous opinions of others who don't understand.
3. Check for a pulse. If you have one . . . you will survive! Believe it.

Dr. Judith Moore

I was thrilled when Marie Osmond first visited me in 1997. She was very open to the integration of both standard and alternative care. I am so grateful that she eventually returned to see me when she was experiencing postpartum depression. This book, which resulted from her visits and treatment at our clinic, will now bless thousands because she was willing to share her very private story.

I consider my most important achievement in life to be motherhood. I am a mother to six children and grandmother to five (so far). I am also a doctor, an osteopathic board-certified family practice physician. An osteopathic physician is trained and licensed in everything a medical doctor is, with the added benefit of learning intimately the structure of the body and how to keep the structure and function of the body working through manual manipulation.

I was a mother before I was a doctor. I started medical school at the age of thirty-five, with my six children ranging in age from three to thirteen. Luckily, I had a supportive husband, who did the best he knew how to be both mother and father when I was not around. I was able to look at my medical training from a different perspective than most young medical students because I had already personally experienced some of what we were taught, especially when it came to pediatrics, obstetrics, and gynecology. My goal was to be a doctor whom women could feel comfortable with because I respected and worked with their feelings.

While training in hospitals in my third year of medical school, I started an internal medicine rotation. The intern I worked with was excellent in internal medicine and taught me a lot. He was also a homeopath and gave me a book to read on the homeopathic philosophy of medicine. The book spoke to my heart and opened my mind to a new way of thinking. Homeopathic physicians look far beyond the disease process to the root cause, which may be physical, emotional, or even spiritual. They consider disease processes at a different level than I had learned. This doctor taught me that I could be an excellent modern physician and also draw from alternative treatments.

I have not abandoned modern medicine, and I can prescribe medicines and recommend surgery as needed, but I also have many other choices to draw from and many viewpoints to look at as I approach a patient.

The Whirlwind:
Marie's First Visit

◆

I received a delightful Christmas gift from Marie: her *Wizard of Oz* porcelain dolls. She told me that she was Dorothy and just wanted to "go home" from this dark hole behind her eyes that she had been in. She told me that I was Glinda, the Good Witch, and the Wicked Witch was PPD. Marie said that all she wanted was a clear brain (the Scarecrow), a loving heart (the Tin Man), and the courage to keep going (the Cowardly Lion), and that she had received these from our office. I was deeply honored by this gift and I display these dolls prominently in my waiting room.

My office staff has commented that Marie's visits are like a whirlwind, similar to Dorothy's tornado in *The Wizard of Oz*. Because she has so many irons in the fire, and because she is frequently traveling, she is not able to come in as often as most of our patients. She is usually whirling in from somewhere out of town, or from an important activity, and while she is at our office, almost the entire staff is involved in discovering all we can about her health and what treatments will work best for her. Then she'll whirl out, scooping up supplements and children, off to her next meeting or event of the day.

Marie's first visit for postpartum depression was on a snowy day in the late fall of 1999. She left Los Angeles, where she was living at the time, early that morning with all her children and flew into Salt Lake City. However, an accident on the freeway slowed their drive from the airport to my office, and she arrived two hours late, at about eleven in the morning. The first words out of her mouth were, "Where is the bathroom?" For one of the tests we were doing, we needed the first urine of the morning. She didn't want to carry the urine on the plane, so she held it in the entire time! We knew right then what a superwoman she was.

After dispatching the precious urine sample, Marie could breathe better, and we gave her a cup to spit in. No, she wasn't chewing tobacco; this was also part of the test. The test we were performing is called a biological terrain assessment (BTA). The BTA tests urine, saliva, and blood to determine acid-alkaline balance, oxidative stress, and electrolyte and mineral concentration.

Marie's test showed that her body was relatively acidic and couldn't balance itself properly because she was losing a lot of minerals in her urine. This was due to her long-standing kidney problems. Minerals are needed, among other things, to keep the body in proper acid-alkaline balance. If the body tissue is too acidic, the cells can't function to full capacity, and eventually fatigue and illness result.

We then obtained a few drops of blood from Marie's finger. Our technician looked at the blood under a high-powered microscope, which was projected on a TV screen so Marie could see it. This test showed that she might have high levels of candida (yeast) in her body. It also showed that she was under possible adrenal stress. Both tests showed that she probably wasn't digesting and absorbing her nutrients well and as a result was malnourished.

We had requested that Marie get some blood tests done in California before she came so we could look at hormone levels and other metabolic processes. There are three kinds of estrogens that the body uses—estradiol, estrone, and estriol. As the fax of her results came in, we found that her estradiol level was on the low end of normal and her estrone level was normal, but her estriol level was very low, and her progesterone level was almost negligible. Her level of DHEA, a hormone precursor, was also low, and her magnesium level was, in my opinion, dangerously low. I explained how each of these problems could contribute to PPD.

We then did an allergy screen on Marie and discovered she was allergic to several foods, food chemical additives, and mold.

With all this information in hand, we put Marie on high doses of natural progesterone, a low dose of DHEA, a course of an anti-fungal medicine for candida, and an allergy-free, sugar-free diet. Marie admitted that she often had little time to eat well while on the set of *Donny & Marie* and would use sugar and chocolate to boost her energy, so we provided a healthy, balanced, soy-based liquid meal substitute for her, called UltraMeal, which would also support her hormones, along with Mega Green, an energy-boosting green drink that would also provide minerals, for her to drink throughout the day. We also provided supplements to combat the deficiencies we found on the tests. We then made plans for her to receive a special allergy shot when she returned after Christmas, to reduce her body's reaction to her environment.

I then started dealing with her pain and muscle spasms using osteopathic manipulative therapy and cranial osteopathy. This is a gentle form of manipulation that allows the connective tissue and muscles to release, which causes improvement in blood, lymph, and nerve flow. While I was working on her, we discussed the importance of dealing with the problems she was facing in her life. I told her that, although I often found depression to be triggered by physical problems, such as hormonal imbalances, it is usually a sign that there are emotional issues that must be dealt with. However, I knew that until her physical problems were improved, it would be difficult for her to deal with the emotional issues.

WHAT IS POSTPARTUM DEPRESSION?

Physical Changes During the Postpartum Period: The Fourth Trimester

Postpartum is the medical term used to describe the period of time following the birth of the baby. Some people call it the "fourth trimester," because so many changes related to the pregnancy are still taking place in the body during this time, both physically and emotionally. These changes are often overlooked and unrecognized in our North American culture, where women are expected to return home from the hospital to a normal routine twenty-four to forty-eight hours after the birth of the baby.

During a woman's pregnancy, her levels of estrogen and progesterone are elevated to many times the normal amount to stimulate placental growth. After the birth, these levels drop rapidly, sometimes to below pre-pregnancy blood levels. These hormonal changes may cause a new mother to experience sweating or hot flashes and hair loss (a woman's hair often becomes thicker during pregnancy; the hair loss after birth usually brings it to a pre-pregnancy state). The increased hormone levels for lactation (prolactin and oxytocin) cause uterine contraction and breast engorgement and have some effect on muscle contraction.

Following birth, the woman's body is working on healing from the trauma of the birth experience. If there has been an episiotomy or tearing requiring stitches, she may be experiencing a lot of discomfort. It may take up to four weeks for the placental site to heal over in the uterus, and bleeding may continue for that time. Fatigue is common as the body heals and replaces blood, and the body needs rest. However, during this time the mother is not able to get much rest, as the baby needs frequent attention. If the birth was cesarean, it may take more than six weeks for the body to completely heal from the surgery.

Even though women are told that intercourse is safe after the six-week checkup, many women find that it is still painful, especially if there was an episiotomy. The hormones for lactation naturally decrease a woman's sexual desire and also may cause vaginal dryness. Because of sleep deprivation and the demands of a new infant, mothers frequently find themselves so exhausted that sexual relations are the last thing on their minds. This may create guilt and stress between partners, adding to the strain of the postpartum period.

Emotional Changes During the Postpartum Period

Up to 80 percent of women experience some degree of "baby blues." This is a feeling of sadness or of being overwhelmed. The new mother may experience mood swings and bouts of crying that begin a few days after the birth of the baby and can last two or three weeks. This is generally thought to be caused by the rapidly changing hormone levels and may be similar to the emotional changes that accompany premenstrual syndrome and menopause. As the hormones level out, the moodiness decreases and eventually dissipates. Typically, the "down" feelings are not constant but come and go, and usually with effort the mother can lift herself out of the blues for a time.

Ten to 15 percent of women go deeper into what is called postpartum depression, or postnatal depression (PPD). PPD usually includes all the symptoms of baby blues, but they are more intense and debilitating, are frequently unrelenting, and do not go away after a few weeks. These symptoms may start as baby blues and continue to intensify, or they may not start for a month or more after the baby's birth. Most often the symptoms are centered on a feeling of "I can't do this" or "I am a terrible mother" or "They would be better off without me." Commonly, there are feelings of inadequacy, guilt, hopelessness, tearfulness, fatigue, and irritability or anger. The symptoms may also include suicidal thoughts or the desire for death, the desire to harm the baby or someone else, irrational fears, anxiety, panic attacks, or obsessive thoughts and compulsions to do repetitive activities, such as the obsessive need for extreme cleanliness or the constant, minute-by-minute compulsion to check on the baby. These feelings rarely let up, and the mother, no matter how hard she works at it, cannot seem to lift herself out of the depression.

In approximately 1 out of 1,000 births, a mother experiences postpartum psychosis. Confusion, fatigue, agitation, delusions, hearing voices or having hallucinations, hyperactivity, not feeling the need to sleep, and rapid speech are symptoms that characterize this disorder. There is usually some loss of touch with reality. There is usually a history of bipolar disorder or previous psychosis in these women, but sometimes this is the first evidence of a problem, as the trauma of the birth, along with hormonal and other physical changes, sets off chemical changes that create the symptoms of psychosis. These symptoms are more severe than PPD and generally signify an emergency. Women experiencing these problems usually need hospitalization and intensive work in order to heal.

QUESTIONNAIRE:
DO YOU HAVE POSTPARTUM DEPRESSION?

This questionnaire is loosely based on the Edinburgh Postnatal Depression Scale, which is used to determine the presence of postpartum depression in research studies. Scores showing a possibility that you have postpartum depression do not prove that you have clinical depression, and I recommend that you visit your OB/GYN or your family practice doctor for a diagnosis.

The following list of possible risk factors for postpartum depression will assist you in responding to the questionnaire.

1. A previous history of clinical depression, anxiety or panic disorder, bipolar disease, eating disorders, or obsessive-compulsive disorder.
2. Poor social support, meaning you have no one you can rely on for assistance or to share intimate thoughts and feelings with.
3. Multiple or serious stressful life events, such as difficulty in family relationships or at work, a recent move, a new job or other major change, the death of a loved one, severe financial problems, or the like.
4. A previous history of severe PMS, menstrual disorders, and/or difficulty becoming pregnant (signs of hormone imbalances).

5. A history of childhood abuse, including emotional, physical, or sexual abuse.
6. Thyroid problems or a family history of thyroid problems.
7. A history of insomnia or excessive sleeping.
8. Chronic or frequent vaginal yeast infections, or frequent antibiotic or steroid use, causing yeast overgrowth in the bowels.
9. A low-fat, low-protein diet, or other poor nutrient diet, or severe morning sickness, which increases malnutrition.
10. A poor relationship with your mother.
11. A mother who had PPD.
12. Oral-contraceptive use or receiving the Depo-Provera shot soon after delivery.
13. Stopping breast-feeding soon after delivery, either by choice or because of lack of adequate milk.
14. High weight gain during pregnancy and/or poor weight loss after pregnancy.
15. A traumatic birth experience, including unexpected cesarean section or the delivery of a preterm infant.
16. Early discharge from the hospital (less than twenty-four to forty-eight hours).

QUESTIONNAIRE:

1. a. My baby is 1 to 7 days in age.
   b. My baby is 8 to 14 days in age.
   c. My baby is 15 to 28 days in age.
   d. My baby is 4 weeks or more in age.
2. a. I have 0–1 risk factors for PPD (see above).
   b. I have 2–3 risk factors for PPD.
   c. I have 4 risk factors for PPD.
   d. I have 5 or more risk factors for PPD.

Next, please mark the answer that comes closest to how you have felt overall during the past seven days, not just how you feel today.

IN THE PAST SEVEN DAYS:

3. I have been able to laugh and see the funny side of things:
   a. As much as I always could.
   b. Not quite so much now.
   c. Definitely not so much now.
   d. Not at all.

4. I have looked forward with enjoyment to things:
   a. As much as I ever did.
   b. Rather less than I used to.
   c. Definitely less than I used to.
   d. Hardly at all.

5. I have blamed myself unnecessarily when things went wrong:
   a. No, never.
   b. Not very often.
   c. Yes, some of the time.
   d. Yes, most of the time.

6. I have felt worried and anxious without a very good reason:
   a. No, not at all.
   b. Hardly ever.
   c. Yes, sometimes.
   d. Yes, very often.

7. I have felt scared or panicky without a very good reason:
   a. No, not at all.
   b. No, not much.
   c. Yes, sometimes.
   d. Yes, quite a lot.

8. I have been feeling overwhelmed:
   a. No; I have been coping as well as ever.
   b. No; usually I have coped quite well.
   c. Yes; sometimes I haven't been coping as well as usual.
   d. Yes; most of the time I haven't been able to cope at all.

9. I have had difficulty sleeping even when the baby is asleep:
   a. No, not at all.
   b. Not very often.
   c. Yes, sometimes.
   d. Yes, most of the time.

10. I have felt sad or miserable:
    a. No, not at all.
    b. Not very often.
    c. Yes, quite often.
    d. Yes, most of the time.

11. I have been so unhappy that I have been crying, or fighting to keep from crying:
    a. No, never.
    b. Only occasionally.
    c. Yes, quite often.
    d. Yes, most of the time.

12. The thought of harming either myself or my baby has occurred to me:
    a. Never.
    b. Hardly ever.
    c. Sometimes.
    d. Yes, quite often.

Scoring:

    a. 0 points
    b. 1 point
    c. 2 points
    d. 3 points

0–8 points: low probability of depression
8–12 points: most likely just dealing with life with a new baby or a case of baby blues
13–14 points: signs leading to the possibility of PPD; take preventive measures as described in the book
15 or more points: high probability of experiencing clinical postpartum depression

Add the points together. A score of 15 or more indicates a probability of postpartum depression. However, this does not confirm the diagnosis, and you should check with your doctor for confirmation. I also recommend that you closely read this book, as you may find information to assist you that your doctor may not know or may not have time to go over with you.

A score of less than 15 does not confirm that you do *not* have PPD. If you have a score of less than 15, the probability is less that this is truly PPD, but if you feel poorly and have concerns, please see your doctor. Even if you do not have a high probability of PPD, the contents of this book may still assist you through your baby blues or other difficult times during your postpartum period.

If you answered either (c) or (d) on question 12, it is imperative that you seek assistance to deal with the possibility, even though you feel that you would never do it, of harming yourself or your baby. Thoughts can build slowly into action, if the thoughts are pervasive enough. Please visit your doctor, or seek the assistance of someone you trust, or call the suicide hotline at 1-800-SUICIDE.

Risk Factors for Postpartum Depression

$$\diamond$$

A PREVIOUS HISTORY OF DEPRESSION

A past history of depression, or feeling depressed during pregnancy, has been shown to increase the risk for PPD. Symptoms may include despondency or despair, feelings of inadequacy, inability to cope, hopelessness, impaired concentration or memory, loss of normal interests, thoughts of death or suicide, thoughts of hurting someone, or other bizarre thoughts. If you have experienced these feelings in the past over an extended period of time, you may have actually had depression, even if a doctor or therapist has not diagnosed you with that condition.

Other emotional diagnoses can also be risk factors for PPD. Anxiety or panic disorder, bipolar or manic-depressive disorder, obsessive-compulsive disorder, or eating disorders such as anorexia nervosa, bulimia, or overeating to appease negative emotions can all be amplified during the postpartum period and can show up in the form of PPD.

Depression can also be manifested by physical symptoms, such as headaches, chest pains, heart palpitations, hyperventilation, or numbness and tingling in the arms or legs. Chronic muscle or joint pain, including the diagnosis of fibromyalgia syndrome, and abdominal pain or digestive upset, including the diagnosis of irritable bowel syndrome, can also be possible signs of depression or emotional stress. All of these symptoms and diagnoses may be caused by other physiologic conditions, such as thyroid problems, candida or other bacterial bowel infection, chronic sinus or tooth infection, food allergies or nutritional deficiencies. However, consider the possibility of severe emotional stress or suppressed depression if a doctor examines you, does appropriate testing, and no real physical diagnosis can be made.

If you are experiencing any of the above, or have experienced them in the past, then you may have an increased risk for PPD and may want to seek assistance to prevent PPD from occurring.

POOR SOCIAL SUPPORT

One hundred years ago most women gave birth to their babies at home. Extended families lived in the same household or close by. A doctor or a midwife attended the birth, along with mothers, aunts, and sisters. These women stayed with or frequently visited the new mother, caring for her and teaching her how to care for the baby.

Fifty years ago, mothers stayed in the hospital for ten days following the birth of the baby. After that, the mother's own mother frequently came to help for another week or two, allowing the new mother to rest during the day when she had been caring for the baby much of the night. This kind of social support has special meaning as new mothers realize that they share with other women common joys and fears, allowing emotional intimacy and connectedness.

Marie's mother was present at the births of her other children and gave her great support. However, Marie told her mother not to stay with her after the birth of Matthew because she was concerned about her mother's health and didn't want to burden her. She didn't realize that the lack of her mother's presence would have such a profound effect upon her.

Studies have shown that women who have very little social support during pregnancy and following delivery have a higher

◆

risk of developing PPD. We all need emotional nourishment, and a new mother, just having completed a traumatic life event that requires her to take on a completely new role, becomes especially vulnerable when her emotional needs are not met.

SUGGESTIONS FOR IMPROVING SOCIAL SUPPORT

1. During your pregnancy, talk with friends and family, and arrange for social support during the first few weeks postpartum, if possible from someone who loves you and wants to take care of you.
2. Arrange to have access to someone with whom you can share your feelings, even if only by telephone. Do these things ahead of time so you don't have to think of what to do when you most need it. Marie admitted that she felt guilty asking anyone for assistance and would turn people down if they offered. She wants to tell you: *Don't feel guilty about asking for assistance.* This is the time in your life when you most deserve it.
3. During your pregnancy, discuss with your partner the anticipated problems of the first few weeks after the baby arrives. Discuss what you feel your needs will be, and encourage a discussion of his fears and needs.
4. If you are not currently experiencing PPD but see signs of PPD in someone you know, seek her out and assist her in whatever way you are able.

MULTIPLE OR SERIOUS STRESSFUL LIFE EVENTS

The stressfulness of life events depends a lot on the meaning we attach to the event. What may be very stressful to one person may create no stress at all in others. There are some events, however, that are generally considered stressful to most people. Remember, a stressful event may be a positive or a negative event; either may create stress. The following is a list of many of these, though not necessarily in order of highest stress, as each event means something different to each individual.

1. Major personal injury or illness, or major surgery, including cesarean section.
2. Death of a spouse.
3. Death of a close family member other than a spouse, or of a close friend.
4. Gaining a new family member (birth, adoption, parent moving in).
5. Major change in the health or behavior of a family member.
6. Buying or building a house, and/or moving to a new residence.
7. Detention in jail or other institution against your will.
8. New job, or major change in job status, or losing a job.
9. Marriage or beginning a new relationship.
10. Marital or relationship problems.
11. Spouse beginning or ending work, or having difficulties at work.
12. A major change in financial situation; money problems.
13. Victim of a major crime.
14. Separation from a spouse.
15. Reconciliation with a spouse.
16. Pregnancy.
17. A child getting married.
18. Vacation.
19. Excessive exercise.
20. Exposure to industrial or environmental toxins.
21. A major change in sleeping habits.
22. A major change in eating habits.
23. A major change in religious or spiritual activities or beliefs.
24. Sexual problems.
25. In-law difficulties.
26. Problems with boss or coworkers.
27. Small children at home.
28. Teenagers at home.

Marie had experienced many of these stressors just before, during, and after her pregnancy. Her high-resolution microscopic blood analysis showed adrenal stress, and she experienced most of the symptoms of relative adrenal insufficiency. If you have experienced several of the stressors listed on the previous page during your pregnancy, your body chemicals may respond, and you may be more susceptible to illness, both physical and emotional.

Cortisol is a hormone that is normally produced by the adrenal glands, small triangular glands that sit on top of the kidneys. Cortisol is frequently called the "stress hormone," as it is produced to assist the body when it is under physical or emotional stress. However, with chronic or excessive stress, the cortisol levels can remain too high, causing problems for the body. Cortisol is a glucocorticoid, or a steroid. The problems related to long-term high levels of cortisol include suppression of the immune system; increased protein breakdown, which leads to muscle wasting and osteoporosis; decrease in the body's ability to make proteins; increased blood pressure; depression; insomnia; suppression of the sex hormones; faster aging; memory loss; increases in blood sugar levels contributing to the development of diabetes, or blood sugar swings causing hypoglycemia; increases in insulin, which increases fat deposition and hardening of the arteries; hypertension; high cholesterol; and binge eating.

Adrenaline is also produced by the adrenal glands during stress. Adrenaline will acutely increase the body's "fight or flight" capacity, increasing heart rate, increasing blood flow to the extremities, releasing blood sugar, and so on. But long-term, chronic adrenaline release can cause increased blood pressure, increased heart rate, insomnia, anxiety, and even panic attacks. The strong feelings of anxiety that Marie felt on her drive to Los Angeles after witnessing the accident were caused by excessive adrenaline.

Another hormone produced by the adrenal gland that is affected by stress is DHEA. DHEA is considered a "mother" hormone, or a building block to many of the sex hormones, including estrogen and testosterone. Lower levels are associated with aging. It also assists the body in stress reactions. Low DHEA levels contribute to the negative effects of high cortisol levels, and the body ages faster and gets sick easier through increased oxidative stress.

Marie was low in DHEA and felt as if her body had aged more during the time she was experiencing PPD.

If a mother's nutrition is poor, or the body is weak from illness, a state of relative adrenal insufficiency can be reached, meaning that the adrenal glands are not able to manufacture the necessary levels of cortisol to keep up with the levels of stress. In this state chronic fatigue sets in, depression becomes worse, blood pressure drops, sugar and insulin levels drop too low, hormone levels change, and the immune system becomes overactive, creating or increasing allergies and, sometimes, autoimmune diseases.

Cortisol levels rise during pregnancy, increase during the third trimester, and reach their highest levels during birth. This is to allow the mother and the infant to handle the stress of the delivery smoothly. A few days after delivery, the body's cortisol levels will generally fall back to their normal, pre-pregnancy state.

However, when the mother has to deal with excessive physical, emotional, and/or mental stress during pregnancy and during the postpartum period, the excessive stress will cause her cortisol levels after delivery to remain abnormally high, with all the attendant problems mentioned above. Adrenaline levels may also remain high, creating anxiety, palpitations, or even panic attacks.

If the mother with excessive stress is already in poor health or has poor nutrition, her body may not be able to make enough cortisol to handle the continued stress during and after delivery, resulting in deep depression, severe fatigue, and the other problems mentioned above. Depression can accompany either one of these conditions, though more often high cortisol is related to an anxious depression and relative low cortisol is related to a deep, fatigue-like depressed state.

Stress Hormone Testing

Tests to ask your doctor about:

Blood cortisol levels—This test is not extremely accurate unless at least four levels are taken during the day and night.

ACTH cortisol stimulation test—This is the test most endocrinologists use to diagnose adrenal insufficiency. This is a more accurate test, but it does not test how well the cortisol is produced over time and during excessive stress.

Saliva stress hormone levels—This test takes four different saliva samples at specific times during the day. My experience has shown that this test is accurate and easy, as the patient can do it at home.

Treatment for Adrenal Stress or Exhaustion

Treatments to ask your doctor about:

Adrenal stress (a chronically elevated cortisol level)—This condition currently has no treatment in Western medicine, unless the diagnosis is Cushing's syndrome, which is usually caused by a tumor; the only treatment available is the removal of the tumor.

Adrenal insufficiency—This is often treated by a doctor with prescription cortisone, or hydrocortisone. If cortisone is given in low doses in order to bring the cortisol levels to normal, this can be an effective treatment and can give the adrenals a rest. These low levels of cortisone have not been shown to harm a nursing baby. However, careful supervision by a doctor is necessary because side effects can be a problem.

Alternative treatments—Both adrenal stress and adrenal insufficiency are treated by feeding the adrenal glands. Ask your doctor if these supplements may be right for you.

1. *Vitamin C*—90 percent of the vitamin C you take in is used by your adrenals.
2. *B complex*—Important in making adrenal hormones. As there is a rapid turnover of these vitamins, and the body quickly excretes any excess, lower doses taken more frequently are useful for feeding the adrenals. Sometimes, if a patient is experiencing digestive problems, such as Marie did, I will give

B complex and B_{12} shots (given by prescription by a doctor) to my patients three times a week for a few weeks while treating the adrenal glands.

3. *Basic multivitamin/mineral*—Many vitamins work better in combination with other vitamins and minerals. A basic multivitamin mineral supplement ensures the basic nutrition necessary to allow the other supplements to work.

4. B_5 (pantothenic acid)—Assists in energy production in the adrenals and elsewhere, and burns excessive cholesterol and triglycerides.

5. B_1 *(thiamine)*—Use extra amounts if your cortisol levels are too high rather than too low.

6. *Magnesium (citrate, glycinate, malate, or fumarate)*—Excretion of magnesium in the urine is increased with high cortisol levels.

7. A good *trace mineral complex,* including manganese and zinc. I like NuLegacy's Colloidal Trace Minerals sublingual drops, which absorb directly under the tongue and don't depend on the digestive system for adequate absorption.

8. *DHEA*—Use only if blood or saliva DHEA levels are too low and if recommended by a doctor, because it is a potent hormone. I use 5–10 mg a day for women, 25–50 mg a day for men, but your doctor may recommend different doses. *Caution:* Do not take this hormone if you have breast, uterine, or, in men, prostate cancer, because DHEA can turn into estrogen and testosterone. Watch for acne, facial hair growth, headaches, stomach problems, and excess mucus as a sign of getting too much DHEA.

9. *Licorice root (glycyrrhiza)*—An excellent treatment to increase your cortisol levels and support your adrenal glands. Some licorice preparations made for ulcers and gastritis have the glycyrrhiza removed. These preparations are not effective for improving adrenal function. *Caution:* Do not use if you have high blood pressure. Signs of getting too much licorice are anxiety or hyperactivity, decreased appetite, heart palpitations, and increased blood pressure.

10. *Progesterone*—If your levels are low, a little natural progesterone cream (1/8 teaspoon a day or less) can provide the body with the base necessary to make cortisol. *Caution:* Do not use if your progesterone levels are high, or if you are hyperthyroid. If you become uncontrollably moody or weepy, or if your periods stop, or you begin to have breakthrough bleeding (bleeding in the middle of your cycle), you may be getting too much progesterone and should cut back on your dosage.

11. *Herbs*—Mullein, lobelia, Siberian ginseng, hawthorn berries, ginger, cayenne. I prefer NuLegacy's ADR Support Plus, which also contains adrenal glandular, and Dr. Christopher's Adrenal Formula (Adrenetone or ADR-NL).

12. *Meditation*—Shown in multiple studies to reduce the effects of stress on the body. Meditation may be more useful than all the supplements combined. There are many good books that describe meditation and the relaxation response. Even fifteen minutes a day of meditation can have a dramatic effect on the body.

13. *Anxiety-reducing nutritional and herbal formulas*—To reduce the effects of stress. I prefer Anxiety Control, made by Pain & Stress Center, which has high levels of GABA, and Dr. Christopher's Nerve Herbal Food Combination (Relax-Eze or MindTrac).

14. When you are feeling stressed out, *stop, look, and listen.* Stop and consider what is bothering you. Look at yourself and observe your emotional state. Listen to your heart to determine if this problem is something worth getting upset over. If it isn't, let it go. If it is, take a moment to experience all the feelings associated with it. Then determine if you can change it. If you can't, let it go. If you can, determine what needs to be done and do it.

15. When you are feeling stressed out, shift your attitude by bringing to your mind someone or something that allows you to *feel unconditional love*—usually a child or a pet—and hold that feeling for at least fifteen seconds. The stress on your body may dramatically drop.

SEVERE PMS, MENSTRUAL DISORDERS, AND/OR DIFFICULTY BECOMING PREGNANT (CAUSED BY HORMONAL IMBALANCE)

A history of premenstrual syndrome, menstrual problems, or infertility is frequently a sign of hormonal imbalance. Often these problems are a sign of relative estrogen dominance and low progesterone. All steroid hormones, including the stress hormone cortisol, are made from cholesterol, and all of them can also be made from progesterone. The body can control deficiencies and excesses of the other hormones by using progesterone. As progesterone is needed to make cortisol, if a new mother is experiencing excessive stress, the progesterone will be used for the cortisol, and DHEA is used to make the other hormones. If the stress continues and the body cannot replenish itself, both progesterone and DHEA levels may drop, as they did in Marie.

Most doctors use synthetic progestins such as Provera. These progestins do not perform many of the functions that the body's own progesterone does. The body's progesterone helps to balance estrogen, is necessary for a normal pregnancy, promotes new bone formation, improves sleep, has a natural calming effect, balances fluids, lowers blood pressure, assists the body in utilizing and eliminating fats, assists with sex drive, improves cholesterol levels, assists in hair growth, and may protect against breast cancer. Marie's progesterone level was extremely low, which caused, among other problems, depression, water retention, weight gain, headaches, and insomnia.

On the other hand, synthetic progestins can suppress your body's own production of progesterone by binding to the progesterone receptors (see page 279). This can create an estrogen-progesterone imbalance, which can lead to fluid retention, weight gain, mood swings, and headaches. If taken during pregnancy, synthetic progestins may cause birth defects. They may also cause blood clots and increase the risk of heart disease and breast cancer.

As mentioned earlier, there are three main types of estrogen: estradiol, estrone, and estriol. Premarin, the most commonly prescribed estrogen, contains estrones and estradiols made from pregnant horses' urine. Estradiol and estrone are very potent, or strong, estrogens, while estriol is considered a weak estrogen and is usually not used in conventional medicine in the U.S. for estrogen replacement. However, estriol is normally found in much larger amounts in the body than are estradiol and estrone and has positive effects on the body.

Estriol is produced in large quantities by the placenta during pregnancy. Estriol is more beneficial to the vagina, vulva, and cervix than the other estrogens and improves post-menopausal urinary tract infections better than estradiol. It seems to have a protective effect, along with progesterone, on proliferation (or tumor formation) of estradiol-sensitive cells, such as are found in the uterus and breast. I frequently find, as I did with Marie, that estrone and estradiol levels are normal in women with PPD, while estriol levels are low.

If you already have a history of hormonal problems going into pregnancy, the hormonal imbalance may become worse after pregnancy, thus increasing your risk of postpartum depression.

Sex Hormone Testing

Blood hormone levels—This is the method that most doctors use. A onetime blood level for hormones looks at the hormones at a moment in time, but hormone levels change throughout the day and throughout the month.

Twenty-four-hour urine sex hormone profile—This test averages the hormone levels over twenty-four hours and tests estradiol, estrone, estriol, progesterone, testosterone, and DHEA. This is a good test for a woman who is not having periods (such as soon after the baby's birth or after menopause).

Twenty-eight-day saliva sex hormone profile—This test is most useful for women who are having periods. It uses saliva samples taken every three days during the cycle. This is the test that most often shows the estrogen dominance and progesterone deficit I find so often with depression, premenstrual syndrome, severe menstrual cramping, excessive menstrual bleeding, fibroids, fibrocystic breast disease, and sometimes endometriosis. It also shows the erratic levels of progesterone that are a sign of adrenal stress or insufficiency. (See the appendix for laboratories that perform the urine and saliva tests.)

Treating Hormones

If your hormonal testing shows:

All hormone levels low—The symptoms may include irregular or no periods, excessive bleeding when you do have a period, fatigue, hot flashes, and emotional changes. This is usually a sign of relative adrenal insufficiency or, if you are the right age, the beginning of menopause. Hormone support during adrenal insufficiency can be provided by either oral contraceptives or natural estriol and progesterone.

Natural hormones are found at compounding pharmacies. They usually need a prescription by a doctor. See the appendix at the back of the book for information on how to find a compounding pharmacist and a physician who will prescribe natural hormones.

Estrogen dominance and/or progesterone deficiency—The symptoms of "unopposed estrogen," which is a high estrogen-to-progesterone ratio, may include sore and/or cystic breasts, periods too close together, heavy bleeding, severe menstrual cramps, hair loss, restlessness, irritability, moodiness, premenstrual syndrome, and insomnia. Often over-the-counter natural progesterone creams such as Pro-Gest can adequately resolve the problem. You want a cream with at least 200 mg of progesterone per ounce. Higher doses of natural progesterone will need a prescription by your doctor.

Elevated progesterone levels (especially during the first half of the cycle)—The main symptoms of this problem are extreme moodiness and possibly breakthrough bleeding, or spotting of blood when it is not time for your period. This is usually a sign of high stress levels, causing adrenal stress. The treatment for adrenal stress is found on page 249.

Herbs for Hormonal Balance

Discuss with your holistic doctor the possible use of herbs for hormonal therapy. Follow your doctor's directions or the directions on the container for the correct dosage. Do not use more than the recommended dosage. Some herbs that your doctor may recommend are:

Chaste tree berry (Vitex agnus castus)—This herb assists the body in balancing the estrogen/progesterone ratio. It is slow acting and may require a period of several months to reach full effect.

Dong quai (Angelica sinensis)—This root has a positive effect on the uterus, lowers blood pressure, and reduces water retention. It may take two weeks to have any effect.

Evening primrose oil—Contains gamma linolenic acid, which assists in regulating the prostaglandins, and has been shown to reduce premenstrual syndrome–type symptoms.

Ginseng (Panax schinseng)—Contains plant hormones, antioxidants, essential fatty acids, and minerals, which assist in balancing hormones and increasing energy. May take several days to affect energy level and two to three weeks to affect hormones.

Wild yam (Dioscorea villosa)—Assists the body in regulating and producing its own natural hormones. Remember that this does not have actual progesterone or estrogen in it, but for many women the herb itself can be very useful.

Recommended herbal formulas—Dr. Christopher's NuFem combined with the formula Changease, NuLegacy's OB-Pro Plus, or PhytoPharmica's FemTone.

A HISTORY OF CHILDHOOD ABUSE, INCLUDING EMOTIONAL, PHYSICAL, OR SEXUAL ABUSE

Childhood abuse is a known risk factor for any kind of depression, including PPD. Sexual abuse victims are four times more likely than the general population to develop a psychiatric disorder. The trauma of childbirth and the subsequent hormonal changes will frequently set off a depression or anxiety that will bring back the trauma of these childhood events. The depression can be deep and severe when it is related to issues of self-worth and shame almost always involved after abuse.

Sometimes the victims of childhood abuse have no memories of the abuse, as trauma to children can be subconsciously repressed. Therefore, if a woman experiences severe postpartum depression that does not resolve with normal treatment, childhood abuse may be one cause to consider, especially if she doesn't remember her childhood well. This can be treated without ever remembering the trauma, but most women, as they are striving to heal, will regain some of the lost memories.

This problem will frequently need specialized treatment by trained therapists and a sympathetic doctor. I also recommend, along with therapy, books that assist you in healing yourself. See the Recommended Reading list at the back of this book.

THYROID PROBLEMS

Thyroid hormone levels rise during delivery and stay elevated for at least twelve hours afterward. This increases the metabolic rate to handle the stress and trauma of delivery and allows the healing processes to function. Levels then return to normal over the next three or four days.

Thyroid problems are more common in the postpartum period than at other times. Because pregnancy is associated with immunosuppressive effects (such as high cortisol levels), a new mother is more likely to experience either hyperthyroidism (overactive thyroid) or hypothyroidism (underactive thyroid) during the postpartum period.

Postpartum thyroiditis is an inflammation of the thyroid that occurs in 5–11 percent of postpartum women and can be a cause of PPD. It usually presents as mild hyperthyroidism one to three months postpartum, followed by mild hypothyroidism. Usually the inflammation completely resolves on its own and the thyroid returns to normal within six to nine months. However, because of the seriousness of the symptoms, medical treatment is usually necessary.

Symptoms of low thyroid (hypothyroidism) may include fatigue, difficulty losing pregnancy weight or weight gain, dry skin, constipation, low body temperature, intolerance to cold, muscle weakness, depression, memory loss, menstrual disorders and hormonal imbalance, infertility, sleep disorders, coarse hair or hair loss, and swelling of hands, feet, and eyelids. Symptoms of high thyroid (hyperthyroidism) may include palpitations, nervousness, feeling hot and sweaty, rapid weight loss, fine tremor, clammy skin, diarrhea, anxiety or depression, and sleep disorders.

Marie had positive thyroid antibodies and had been on thyroid medication for years. However, Marie's tests at her first visit showed lower levels of thyroid hormone than are optimum. We changed the type of thyroid medication she was taking, and her levels improved.

Thyroid Testing

Blood thyroid function tests—The testing most doctors use.

Saliva thyroid function tests—These may be more accurate than blood levels, as they measure the biologically active levels of the hormones. Many physicians are not aware that this type of testing is available. See the appendix for laboratories that do this type of testing.

Testing thyroid function by basal body temperature—Test your temperature with a glass thermometer. The testing should be done before getting out of bed in the morning, so the thermometer will need to be placed next to the bed the night before. The most accurate form of testing is under the arm for ten minutes; however, I find good results with testing for five minutes under the tongue. Testing should be for at least three mornings, with an average taken. If the average oral temperature is 97.5 degrees Fahrenheit or below, a low dose of thyroid medication prescribed by your doctor may improve your symptoms. Both blood and temperature testing should be repeated in six weeks to ensure that the patient is getting enough thyroid medication or is not getting too much, which causes hyperthyroid symptoms and suppresses the thyroid gland function.

INSOMNIA OR EXCESSIVE SLEEPING

Insomnia can be defined as difficulty going to sleep and/or difficulty staying asleep, so that the lack of sleep affects your daytime well-being. A history of insomnia can increase your risk for PPD.

Insomnia can be a sign of depression, especially when one wakens early in the morning and has difficulty going back to sleep. Insomnia can also be a sign of anxiety, particularly evidenced when busy thoughts and worries keep one from falling asleep. Insomnia can be a sign of low serotonin, low melatonin (caused by lack of light, aging, or tryptophan deficiency), high cortisol (from high stress), hormonal imbalance, or thyroid imbalance. It is important that you see a doctor to be evaluated for any physical or psychological condition that could be affecting your sleep.

Foods, supplements, and medications that contain caffeine (including chocolate), ephedrine, amphetamine, tobacco, or alcohol can cause insomnia (yes, alcohol may help you go to sleep, but it can cause early waking).

Excessive sleep or sleepiness may also be signs of PPD. They can be caused by depression, low cortisol levels, thyroid imbalances, and sex hormone imbalances, which can each increase the risk of postpartum depression. They can also be caused by hypoglycemia, mononucleosis, chronic fatigue syndrome, allergies, and chronic infections such as sinusitis or tooth infections. High-carbohydrate meals and certain supplements and medications may also cause sleepiness. A need for unusual amounts of sleep or excessive daytime sleepiness should be evaluated.

Sleep loss in the first few months of motherhood can add up to physical, mental, and emotional difficulties. Sleep loss accumulates, and new mothers may carry a dangerously large sleep debt.

With excessive loss of sleep, neurotransmitters are affected and mood deteriorates first, resulting in irritability and sadness. Sleep debt can inhibit immune cells called natural killer-cells, thereby increasing the risk of infection and other diseases. Job performance drops, with more difficulty concentrating and remembering. The number of car accidents doubles among the sleep-deprived, mental functions decline, judgment fades, and critical decisions become difficult to make.

Marie's baby, Matthew, was quite fussy and demanded a lot of her sleep time. Occasionally Marie purposely stayed awake at night to spend time and play with Matthew when she wasn't with him during the day. However, she was also experiencing insomnia because of both physical and emotional problems, so that even when she tried to sleep, she couldn't. The sleep deprivation became severe and added to the severity of her depression.

If it is only a wakeful baby that causes the lack of sleep, depression can be lifted by simply having someone else take responsibility for the baby for a night, allowing the mother to get a good night's sleep. However, if the lack of sleep resulting from a wakeful newborn is combined with insomnia from other factors, these other factors need to be addressed before the new mother can feel well again.

Here are some tips that may assist you in your quest for a good night's sleep:

1. Cut out of your diet all caffeine (coffee, tea, caffeinated sodas, chocolate, and medications with caffeine), alcohol, and tobacco. Caffeine and tobacco are stimulants and can affect

sleep, and alcohol, even though a sedative, will cause early waking as its effect wears off. Often, cutting out caffeine alone will cure the insomnia! Be aware that each of these substances is addictive, and as you eliminate them, the body will go through a withdrawal process, meaning you will generally feel worse before you feel better. A doctor's assistance with withdrawal is often useful.

2. Check out your room—make sure your mattress and pillows are clean, comfortable, and not causing allergies due to dust, dust mites, or feathers. Ensure that your room is completely dark—get heavy curtains or shades if there is a lot of light outside. Determine if the room is noise-free—even a ticking clock can keep some people awake.

3. Put the clock where you can't see it. Clock watching induces anxiety.

4. If you are not able to fall asleep, go to bed an hour later or get up an hour earlier on a regular basis. If you do not expect as much sleep, much of your anxiety about not sleeping will diminish, and sometimes that alone will resolve your problem.

5. If you are not sleeping, stop trying to sleep. Trying to sleep brings on anxiety that keeps you from sleeping. Don't be afraid of not sleeping. Accept the fact that you are not sleeping, and do something to distract your mind, such as reading or listening to quiet music.

6. Counting sheep is not a bad idea. Or concentrate on your breathing and count your breaths. This keeps your mind from being distracted by multiple thoughts and allows it to go into a relaxation state that is very restful. This relaxation can often be as effective as sleeping.

7. Sleepless nights may be a sign of an unresolved issue that is important to deal with. Use the sleepless time to deal with issues you don't have time to think about during the day. Consider what the problem may be, and ponder, meditate, or write about it, rather than worrying. Often sleep will return when the problem is acknowledged.

8. If you nap during the day, a ten-minute nap is more effective than a thirty-minute nap or longer in producing an immediate and sustained recovery in alertness, mood, and performance. A longer nap also increases the risk that you will not sleep again that night.

Natural Supplements for Insomnia

If none of the above works adequately, consider using these natural supplements to assist you in falling asleep. Check with your holistic doctor to see if these would work for you and what dosages to use.

Melatonin—This is a hormone made by the pituitary gland that helps the body become tired and induces sleep. It can be very effective, and most people who use it feel better. However, a small number of people may become depressed using melatonin, so be aware of how you are feeling when you use it. Melatonin can also suppress the growth hormone if used extensively, so children should not use it.

Homeopathic remedies

1. *Coffea crudum*—Homeopathic coffee improves sleep in people whose minds remain very active or who are restless and can't lie still when they are trying to sleep.
2. *Ignatia*—Useful for people who can't sleep because of emotional shock or trauma, or if they are very tired and yawn a lot but cannot sleep, or if they dread going to sleep and have nightmares.
3. *Nux vomica*—Useful for those who overwork, have great mental strain, or overindulge in stimulants, food, or alcohol. Lack of sleep usually makes them irritable.
4. *Gelsemium*—Useful for sleeplessness when you are anticipating all that needs to be done the next day, or when you are feeling achy or have flulike symptoms. This is my husband's favorite sleep remedy.

Herbal remedies—My favorite is Dr. Christopher's Slumber, which contains black cohosh, capsicum, hops, lobelia, skullcap, valerian, wood betony, and mistletoe. This combination lessens the irritability and excitement of the nervous system.

YEAST INFECTIONS

If you experience frequent vaginal yeast infections, have a history of frequent or long-term antibiotic use (such as for infections or acne), have a history of frequent or long-term steroid use (such as for asthma or arthritis), use prescription estrogen or birth control pills, or have frequent or chronic fungal skin infections, you may have an overgrowth of candida or other yeast forms in your bowel and elsewhere in your body. High levels of yeast in the body will increase the risk of PPD.

Some of the symptoms associated with yeast overgrowth are excessive gas and bloating, frequent constipation or diarrhea, sore and/or white tongue, sugar cravings, difficulty concentrating and remembering, mood swings and depression, allergy symptoms, fatigue, muscle aches, numbness or tingling in the hands and feet, an increased number of viral and bacterial infections, and hormonal imbalances. We do not yet have complete knowledge as to how yeast affects the body to create all these symptoms, but they frequently improve when we treat for yeast overgrowth.

If your nursing baby gets thrush (a thick white or white-yellow coating on the tongue and possibly on the roof of the mouth) or a yeast-caused diaper rash, this is a candida infection. Consider the possibility that the baby may have gotten the infection from you. I generally recommend treating both the mother and the baby for candida when a nursing baby has thrush or a yeast-caused diaper rash; however, you should obtain the advice of your own doctor on this issue.

Treatment for Yeast Overgrowth

My partner, Dennis Remington, M.D., is an expert in the candida syndrome and has written a book called *Back to Health: A Comprehensive Medical and Nutritional Yeast Control Program*, which describes in detail the problems and symptoms related to yeast overgrowth and treatments for it. If you think that yeast overgrowth may be a problem for you, I highly recommend this book. It also has a section for physicians if you find that your doctor is interested.

Treatment generally consists of a diet avoiding sugar, fruit, yeast, cheese, and foods that turn quickly into sugar, as yeast feeds off sugar. A good probiotic, which is a supplement that contains the normal "good" bacteria found in the colon, is taken three times a day. If the infection is chronic, often prescription medications are needed, such as nystatin, Nizoral, Diflucan, Sporonox, or other systemic antifungal medication. Some natural products that may reduce the amount of yeast and fungus include, among others, caprylic acid, undecylenic acid, garlic, oregano oil, citrus-seed extract, and pau d'arco. Combination products I use often are NuLegacy's Colloidal EraDeTox, which absorbs under the tongue, and NuLegacy's Candida Pro-Zyme, which is taken with meals and also aids in digestion.

A POOR DIET OR SEVERE MORNING SICKNESS

A poor diet will often result in depression, and a poor diet before, during, and/or after pregnancy can increase the risk of postpartum depression.

The typical American diet may create problems for many women. Marie admitted during her visits to my clinic that her schedule made it very difficult for her to fix and eat healthy meals, and during her pregnancy and postpartum period her diet was often processed and fast foods, with chocolate for energy. The typical American diet today is made up mostly of white flour and sugar. Vegetables are often neglected except in the form of a simple salad, which is often not high in nutrients. Many processed foods are full of sugar and chemicals with very little nutritional value. Excessive sugar and many food additives interfere with the absorption and utilization of nutrients. Most of the processed foods contain man-made hydrogenated fats that interfere with the utilization of good fats in the body.

A major problem with the modern diet is poor mineral absorption and utilization. Minerals are needed for almost every chemical process in the body. Processed foods tend to be low in minerals and high in simple carbohydrates. The body breaks these carbohydrates down quickly into sugar. The excess sugar upsets the electrolyte, or acid-base, balance in the system, causing increased acidity in the tissues. When the body is overly acidic, minerals are utilized to bring the body back into balance, and if minerals are deficient, the body remains acidic. Deficiencies in various trace minerals can also have an effect on mood.

One very important mineral is magnesium. Eating sweets and white sugar, white flour, and white rice can deplete magnesium. Excessive stress depletes magnesium. Diuretics deplete magnesium. A magnesium deficit can cause chocolate cravings. A magnesium deficit can also cause cardiac arrhythmias, chronic muscle spasms, bladder spasms, menstrual cramps, asthma, migraine, irritable bowel, depression, fatigue, insomnia, panic attacks, hypertension, and, if severe, sudden death.

Magnesium is given intravenously in women with toxemia of pregnancy to reduce their high blood pressure. I believe many cases of toxemia are caused by a magnesium deficit. It is hard for physicians to see a magnesium deficiency unless it is very severe. Vitamin B_6 is needed to utilize magnesium in the body, and pregnant women also tend to have a vitamin B_6 deficit, as evidenced by the nausea of pregnancy and increased rates of carpal tunnel syndrome during pregnancy. Marie's blood level of magnesium was abnormally low, meaning her deficiency was severe. She had many of the symptoms described above, including severe muscle spasms. I believe that the severely painful muscles spasms that took Marie to the emergency room a week after Matthew was born were caused by magnesium deficiency.

Most women who experience morning sickness often eat a high-simple-carbohydrate, low-protein diet, and may also eat a low-fat diet, as these foods seem to reduce the nausea. When the nausea of pregnancy becomes severe, there may be very few foods that the mother-to-be can keep down. If the nausea and vomiting last only a few weeks, the mother's body will usually recover, but if the nutritional status remains poor over an extended period of time, either through lack of eating or constant vomiting, then the risk of PPD increases.

I will often have women come into my office complaining of a triad of symptoms: fatigue, hormonal problems, and depression. These women are baffled, as they have been carefully watching their diets and eating what is considered very healthy food. As I take their diet histories, I learn that most of these women have been eating a high-carbohydrate, low-fat, low-cholesterol, and low-protein or even vegetarian diet. The medical community has espoused this diet for two decades now as the best diet for heart disease, and it does work well for some people. However, for many people, especially women, their interpretation of this diet needs a closer look, for the following reasons:

1. I find that women do better when their cholesterol level is between 150 and 200. One of the most important functions of cholesterol is to make hormones. Cholesterol is the building block of progesterone, DHEA, testosterone, and the estrogens. If the body does not have enough cholesterol to work with, the hormone levels may be low.

   Cholesterol also is the building block of the steroid cortisol, the stress hormone. If a person is under a lot of stress, the available cholesterol preferentially goes to the production of cortisol. A study of race car drivers showed that their cholesterol levels dramatically increased after the race and remained elevated for several weeks. Elevated cholesterol levels can be caused by stress. Low cholesterol levels may decrease the amount of cortisol available to respond to stress.

Aldosterone is another chemical made from cholesterol. It affects, among other things, fluid levels in the body, and decreased levels can decrease blood pressure and be a factor in chronic fatigue syndrome.

2. If the blood triglyceride level is below 100 I become concerned. The brain is made of 60 percent fats, and good fats are necessary for proper brain function. A layer of fatty acids makes up the membrane that surrounds every cell in the body. Brain and nerve cells need specific fatty acids to maintain their health. People with deficiencies in the omega-3 and omega-6 fatty acids tend to have difficulty focusing, learning, and remembering and tend to be depressed. A very low fat diet has been found in studies to compromise immune function and increase the infection rate. Good fats also are important in reducing inflammation and hardening of the arteries and assisting many other vital functions.

3. Low-protein diets can, among other things, affect neurotransmitter levels. Neurotransmitters are chemicals that carry messages between brain cells and nerve cells and take these messages throughout the body. One of the best-known neurotransmitters that affect mood is serotonin. Serotonin is made from tryptophan, an amino acid found in many protein foods. Serotonin is a calming neurotransmitter, which allows you to feel relaxed and optimistic. It allows you to be creative and focused. You need adequate serotonin to be able to fall asleep and sleep deeply. The effects of low serotonin seem to be depression, short attention span, poor focusing and organizational skills, acting impulsively, insomnia, and craving sweets and breads. Many of the antidepressant prescription drugs are based on increasing serotonin levels in the body.

Studies have shown that when someone eats a high-carbohydrate meal, especially a meal high in sugar and bread, tryptophan is absorbed in higher amounts by the brain cells. This causes an increase in serotonin levels, resulting in a lifting of mood. Sugars, chocolate, and simple carbohydrates also increase the levels of endorphins, the body's own opiate-like "feel good" drug. When people crave sugars, chocolate, and breads, they are often self-medicating to lift their mood.

However, when a person is eating mostly carbohydrates and very little protein and fat, depression can become worse. Protein is needed to provide tryptophan and other raw materials to make serotonin and to keep the brain healthy. On a low-protein diet, eventually the body may run low on tryptophan, so that the sugary foods elevate the mood for only a short time but can cause a worsening of depressive and other symptoms soon after eating.

Protein also assists in keeping the blood-sugar levels stable. Protein and good fats eaten along with carbohydrates slow down the digestion and absorption of the carbohydrates, causing a more steady release of simple sugars into the bloodstream. Adequate levels of protein and fat are also necessary to keep insulin levels stable. A normal insulin level helps mood, reduces obesity, and improves the overall general health of the body.

Recommended Diet

The diet I most often recommend for general good health during and after pregnancy is as follows. If you have a chronic illness or special needs, consult your doctor before changing your diet.

1. Eat natural, whole foods whenever possible. Any processing reduces the nutrient value.
2. Eat at least four to five servings of fresh (or possibly frozen, especially in the winter) vegetables a day (and I don't count iceberg lettuce as a vegetable because it contains few nutrients). Eat at least two or three servings of green or leafy vegetables a day and at least one orange or yellow vegetable. Vegetables are high in minerals and vitamins and provide carbohydrates and some protein. They assist in reducing excess

acidity in the tissues, bringing the body into a better acid-base balance. It has been shown time and again—people who eat the most vegetables have less cancer and tend to be healthier in every respect. Eat one to three of your vegetable servings raw. The raw plants contain enzymes that assist in digestion and toxin breakdown. Wash your vegetables well to remove pesticides and bacteria.

3. Eat two or three servings of fresh fruit a day. Eat them with other foods as much as possible to slow the absorption of sugars. Fresh fruit is a good source of quick energy, and full of enzymes, minerals, vitamins, and fiber. As much as possible eat fruits that are currently in season, as their nutrient value is much higher. The whole fruit is preferable to the fruit juice, unless you are ill and trying to get extra nutrition in. A glass of orange juice contains the juice of approximately six oranges, which contains a lot of nutrition but also a lot of fruit sugar. Reserve fruit juices for when you really need the extra nutrition. Do not eat fruit if you have a candida (yeast) infection.

4. Eat grains, seeds, and legumes in their whole form as much as possible, rather than processed in flour and breakfast cereals. Nuts and seeds should be eaten raw, and grains can be eaten raw if they are sprouted. When cooked, grains should be soaked for twelve to twenty-four hours and cooked over very low heat for several hours to maintain their enzymes.

5. Eat enough protein. What constitutes "enough" protein is a controversial issue at this time, but I usually recommend a palm-size piece of protein (meat, fish, cheese, soy, or eggs) at each meal, especially if you suspect that you may have high insulin levels, resulting in low or high blood sugar. A bigger person will have a bigger palm and will use more protein than a small person. A person who exercises heavily, such as an athlete in training, may need more protein; however, larger amounts of protein, the size of a steak covering the plate, are not necessary and may be harmful. A person who is careful about food combining may do extremely well as a vegetarian, but I usually do not recommend that pregnant and nursing

mothers follow a vegetarian diet unless they are completely committed to getting adequate protein through carefully combining proteins and eating a wide variety of vegetables, grains, legumes, and fruits. Eggs are a good source of protein and other nutrients. Eat fresh or frozen (not breaded or processed) fish several times a week for the essential oils and iodine. And I do suggest that you eat red meat several times a week, to keep iron and vitamin B_{12} levels adequate. I believe that you need not worry about cholesterol levels, because if you follow this diet faithfully, elevated cholesterol levels should drop.

6. Do not skip meals. In fact, try not to go longer than three or four hours without eating. Your body functions much better on smaller meals eaten more frequently. This will allow your body to let go of fat more easily by stabilizing insulin levels. Eat healthy snacks, such as nuts and seeds, avocados, raw vegetables, and cheese.

7. Reduce sugar (sucrose, dextrose, corn syrup, et cetera) intake to two or three times a week rather than several times a day. Cut out sugary cereals, snacks, and sugar drinks, and eat sugar only as a special-occasion dessert, and just after a meal. If you are trying to lose weight or improve your health, cut out sugar altogether. If you have diabetes, hypoglycemia, symptoms suggestive of a candida (yeast) problem, or suspect a sugar allergy, sugar should be avoided entirely with few exceptions. If you have sugar cravings, be sure to eat high-protein snacks often, and use the amino acid L-glutamine, which will feed your brain and reduce the cravings. Buffered vitamin C with calcium may also reduce sugar cravings.

8. Reduce flour product use (bread, cereals, pasta) to once a day. This will dramatically reduce your processed-food intake, and you will be surprised at how well you feel as you increase your nutrients through whole grains and other foods. Reduction of flour intake will also assist in reducing insulin levels and in maintaining appropriate blood-sugar levels. If you are trying to lose weight, cut out flour products altogether for a

few months. You will lose weight much faster and will feel much better. Frequent high-protein snacks and the amino acid L-glutamine mentioned on the previous page may also reduce bread cravings.

9. Drink at least two quarts of water (preferably filtered or reverse-osmosis-treated water to remove chlorine and other chemicals) a day. Spring and deep well water, if proven uncontaminated, are also acceptable. Distilled water is pure and has no chlorine or toxic compounds but also has no minerals. If you drink distilled water, be sure that you get enough minerals from other sources. Do not drink softened water. If you are experiencing any disease, drink greater amounts of water. This is above and beyond any other beverage you drink, though I would reduce any other beverage, even fruit juice and milk, to one or two glasses a day. If you juice vegetables, you may drink as much as you wish.

10. Use good oils in your cooking and salad dressings, such as olive oil, walnut oil, grape-seed oil, safflower oil, sunflower oil, and canola oil.

11. Avoid aspartame (NutraSweet) and other artificial sweeteners, which some authorities believe can be toxic (see *The Truth About Artificial Sweeteners* by Dennis Remington, M.D.). Also avoid caffeinated beverages, carbonated beverages, alcohol, fried foods (except when fried in good oils), and hydrogenated oils, such as margarine and vegetable-based fats like Crisco. These foods all put excess stress on the body, create toxins, and block or utilize extra nutrients. Avoid additives such as preservatives and MSG, and clean vegetables and fruits to remove pesticides and bacteria. Soaking them in vinegar and water will help.

12. Consider food allergies if you feel worse after a meal, or if you have chronic nasal congestion or sinusitis, asthma, ADD, irritable bowel syndrome, excessive gas, bloating, diarrhea or constipation, difficulty losing weight, or other chronic, unexplained symptoms. Depression, including PPD, can be aggravated by eating foods you may have an allergy to. See the

appendix for laboratories that do food allergy testing, or follow an elimination diet: Don't eat diary products, wheat, corn, citrus fruits, peanuts, sugar, or food coloring and preservatives for ten to fourteen days. Then add the foods back into your diet one at a time, eating several servings of the food during the day, and watch your symptoms over the next twenty-four hours. If one or more of your symptoms worsens, you will know which food is affecting you.

13. Balance your foods and find what works best for you. Many people feel their best on a "40-30-30" type of diet: 40 percent of calories from carbohydrates, 30 percent of calories from proteins, and 30 percent of calories from good fats. This balance is especially useful for people with diabetes, hypoglycemia, hypertension, high blood-lipid levels, high insulin levels, and obesity that doesn't respond to a low-fat diet. Other people feel best on higher levels of healthy carbohydrates and lower amounts of protein, and some feel best as vegetarians. Everyone's body is different and there is no one diet that is best for everyone. Work until you find what gives you the best energy and allows you to feel healthy.

14. Never say never. When we deny ourselves a food, we may soon binge on it. If occasionally you find you cannot resist a certain food that may be on the "no, no" list, sit down and really enjoy it. Let go of the guilt. The guilt from eating a "forbidden" food is worse for the body than the food is. Let yourself plan for and enjoy a special meal once in a while without feeling as if you have "blown it."

RELATIONSHIP WITH AND HISTORY OF YOUR MOTHER

A Poor Relationship with Your Mother

It has been shown through studies that poor bonding or a poor relationship between the new mother and her own mother increases the risk of postpartum depression.

While Marie has a good relationship with her mother, she was unable to connect with her after Matthew's birth. Marie's mother was experiencing her own health problems, and Marie felt guilty about burdening her, so she would always tell her mother that she was "fine."

If you have a strained relationship with your mother, find ways to work through your feelings, through counseling or otherwise, so that you may heal this relationship, if possible, or at least find peace concerning it. If your mother is not available to connect with, either because of death, poor health, or a poor relationship, work on finding a mother substitute among friends or other relatives.

A Mother Who Had Postpartum Depression

Whether through genetics or learned behavior, a new mother whose own mother experienced postpartum depression is at greater risk of experiencing it herself. Talk with your mother and discuss what feelings she may have experienced after the births of her babies. Marie's mother had also experienced postpartum depression, as Marie discovered after her trip up the coast.

OTHER HORMONAL ISSUES: CONTRACEPTIVE USE AND BREAST-FEEDING

Oral Contraceptive Use, or Receiving a Progestin Injection Soon After Delivery

One small study was done in England concerning women who received an injection of progestin for birth control after delivery. This group of women showed an increased incidence of postpartum depression over those that did not receive any hormones for birth control. This may be because the synthetic progestins cause a relative progesterone deficiency. I did not find any studies on oral contraceptive use, but in my own experience I have seen some women become depressed on certain types of birth control pills, and the depression stopped when they stopped taking them. However, many women do well on birth control pills and experience no problems whatsoever.

If you are depressed and are using hormonal contraception, and nothing else seems to be helping, you may want to stop using the hormones for a month to see if the synthetic hormones are worsening the condition.

Stopping Breast-feeding Soon After Delivery, Either by Choice or Because of Lack of Adequate Milk

Prolactin is the hormone that causes the production of breast milk. Prolactin levels increase during pregnancy, but the high levels of estrogens and progesterone at that time inhibit the production of milk. When estrogen and progesterone levels decrease to normal levels after delivery, prolactin can then stimulate the production of milk. Oxytocin, a hormone that is produced by the baby's suckling at the breast, allows the letdown of milk into the breasts. The increased level of oxytocin also stimulates the production of prolactin. Therefore, the more the baby sucks, the more prolactin is produced.

It has been shown in studies of hormone levels in the postpartum period that women with postpartum depression often have lower levels of prolactin than nondepressed women. Lower prolactin levels may decrease the amount of milk available and cause the mother to stop nursing. Because prolactin levels rise during stress, excessive stress may drain the body of the prolactin available and may be one reason prolactin levels eventually become too low, resulting in postpartum depression.

Marie's milk supply was too low to sustain her baby, and she started supplementing within a few days of his birth. She most likely had prolactin levels that were too low to keep her milk production up.

If you find yourself with low levels of breast milk that cannot sustain your baby, see the referrals in the appendix to find assistance with ways to increase your milk supply.

Another study showed that women who chose not to breast-feed their babies had higher rates of postpartum depression than those who did breast-feed. When a woman does not breast-feed her baby, her prolactin levels decrease. It is not known whether the prolactin itself has mood-changing properties or whether the lack of the bond created by nursing contributes to depression. I recommend a woman breast-feed at least three months, if possible. If a mother is working, pumping the milk will keep the prolactin levels adequate.

WEIGHT GAIN

Marie found it very difficult after Matthew's birth to lose some of the weight gained during her pregnancy. Studies have shown that women who perceive themselves to be overweight during their postpartum period have an increased risk of postpartum depression. There is usually some fat deposition in the lower abdomen that comes with each pregnancy and doesn't go away. Excessive stress during and after pregnancy can also cause obesity and affect PPD. See page 267 for suggestions for a healthy diet that can assist weight loss.

A TRAUMATIC BIRTH EXPERIENCE

Studies have shown that women who have a traumatic childbirth experience, including unexpected cesarean section, or give birth to an infant with problems, such as a preterm infant who must remain in the hospital, have higher rates of postpartum depression. A birth experience that goes contrary to what a mother expects can also increase the risk. Marie was expecting her baby to come the first time she was put on Pitocin in California. It was extremely disappointing when labor did not progress after many hours of contractions. After that, as days went by and there was still no sign of labor, the stress of the commitments Marie had made for the upcoming season of *Donny & Marie* began to weigh heavily on her mind, and she chose to be induced again.

A homeopathic remedy to ask your holistic doctor about if you are grieving from trauma or loss, or are experiencing unfulfilled expectations concerning the birth, is ignatia, a microdose of the herb St. Ignatius bean. This remedy will often assist in bringing calm and greater acceptance to the mother.

THE FATHER'S EXPERIENCE OF LIVING WITH POSTPARTUM DEPRESSION

No one except the mother herself is more affected by PPD than the father or partner. Mothers in the midst of their dark hole describe feeling overwhelmed, burdened with responsibility, and completely alone, and believe that no one else can understand them. They withdraw into themselves and stop communicating. The majority of mothers with PPD experience a loss of sexual desire. These symptoms often alter a couple's relationship to the point where the father feels bewildered as to what is happening to the mother and what he should do about it.

Many fathers are not even aware that PPD exists, and few understand the condition and how to best support their depressed spouse. A full 10 to 15 percent of new fathers will experience PPD with their partner and are themselves at higher risk of becoming depressed.

Fathers report that most often, there are no symptoms of depression in the woman before the delivery of the baby. Following the baby's birth and the onset of depression, however, they notice that their wife's behaviors, ways of relating, and personality significantly change. They report that they often feel as if they are living with a new person whom they no longer know how to relate to. The ways of interaction that worked before no longer work, and the most common reaction from fathers at the beginning of depression is confusion, fear, and concern. They often fear that the change is permanent and wonder if their spouse will ever be the same again.

In the beginning, the father has a strong need to fix the problem. Something is wrong with his family and he feels a heavy responsibility to make it right again. Many will take over household duties and care of the infant and other children to make their spouse feel better. Over time, though, the fathers begin to see that they have no control over the situation, and that they cannot fix the problem no matter what they do.

Fathers often become exhausted, overwhelmed, and depressed. They describe their world as collapsing around them. Their increased and sometimes heroic effort is often unappreciated by their spouse or anyone else. Many start feeling anger and resentment, and then are upset at themselves because they know their wife is unable to control the PPD. They end up feeling as if no one understands them. The one person they would normally go to with their problems is withdrawn and distant, and may even be blaming them for much of the problem.

Fathers begin to feel trapped. They dread going home because they never know what to expect from their spouse. There may be a few good days, followed by some very bad ones. Many are afraid to leave their spouse alone for fear that she might harm herself or the baby or be unable to care for the baby. Others express fear of potential suicide. The fathers often refuse out-of-town trips for their work, call home frequently, or have family and friends check up on the mother frequently. Some report that their wives will frequently call them at work requesting that they come home.

One of the biggest problems husbands and partners face is the loss of intimacy, the loss of the way things had once been, both emotionally and sexually. Many men feel unloved after being rejected day after day.

Many fathers become depressed themselves at some point during their spouse's PPD. Factors that put fathers at greater risk for depression are being unemployed, relationship problems with their spouse even before the PPD, less education, a high number of stressful life events, and poor social support.

What Can Dad do?

1. Read this book. Your spouse may be unable to make the effort or concentrate enough to find the assistance she needs from the information here. Note the problems that may be similar to your wife's. Let her know that she is not alone in her suffering and that there are reasons for it.

2. Don't be afraid. Receive counseling or other emotional work together. If you have had relationship problems even before the PPD, make sure these are addressed as soon as possible, or the marriage may not survive the PPD.

3. Don't use anger. Do not take your spouse's anger or emotional and physical withdrawal personally. She usually does not know why she is acting the way she is and has little control over it. Do not interpret this as a sign that she does not love you. Take time to feel your emotional reactions to what is happening, preferably in private or with a counselor.

4. Find social support. Make an effort to find social support other than your spouse. Develop friendships and activities that can lift you when life becomes too hard. Take a little time for yourself. Get a baby-sitter.

5. Ask for assistance. If you find yourself feeling depressed, seek help. Depression in men is often manifested by increased irritability or anger; withdrawing from the family through work, TV, alcohol, or outside activities; an increased need to control others; sleep disturbances; and a feeling of being trapped. If you see any of these signs in yourself, talk to a doctor or counselor about them.

6. Continually express love. Tell your spouse that you love her no matter how she is acting and what problems she may be having, that you are blessed to have her as your wife in any and every situation. She may not seem to hear or react, but a part of her heart will hear it, and if it is said often enough, and acted upon, she will believe it, and you will too!

7. IT WILL END! Remember that the great majority of PPD cases resolve over time. Just knowing that it will end makes it easier to bear.

TREATMENT FOR POSTPARTUM DEPRESSION

Now that you have determined that you may have postpartum depression, what can be done? If you have a knowledgeable and sympathetic doctor, following his or her advice may give you the best results. Review the risk factors for postpartum depression, consider those problems that you have the highest probability of having, and ask for the tests that are most likely to diagnose those problems. See the appendix for names of laboratories that perform some of the specialty testing your doctor may not be familiar with.

Laboratory Tests for Postpartum Depression

The list below includes the most significant laboratory tests.

Sex hormone levels—Estradiol, estrone, estriol, progesterone, testosterone, DHEA (see page 253).

Thyroid function testing—To check for overactive or underactive thyroid function (see page 257).

Complete blood count (CBC)—To check for anemia or infection.

Metabolic panel—To check for electrolyte imbalances, acid-base imbalances, calcium levels, lipid levels, and protein levels.

Magnesium level—Lower levels are more frequent in PPD (level should be around 2.0) (see page 264).

Stress hormone profile—Saliva cortisol and DHEA levels four times during a twenty-four-hour period (see page 248).

High-resolution microscopic blood cell analysis—This test is not available through most physicians and must be performed by a well-trained physician or technician. The test process consists of looking at a drop of blood through a high-powered microscope, which is often projected onto a TV monitor so the patient as well as the technician can see the results of the test. This allows the physician to visualize the basic condition of the blood and to then use this information for specific treatments or as a guide to further testing.

Biological terrain assessment—This test is not available through most physicians. It is a test utilizing blood, urine, and saliva to determine, among other things, the acid-base balance of the body, and can determine which systems of the body are under stress. This can lead to specific diet and supplement recommendations.

Antidepressant Medications: Will They Work for You?

The symptoms of depression are often relieved by use of these drugs, sometimes quite dramatically. However, some patients experience side effects such as fatigue and what I call "mental numbness." In this mental numbness, the extremes of both negative *and positive* feelings are suppressed; this was what Marie found so difficult to live with when she tried antidepressant medication.

Most people feel relief as they start antidepressant medication. However, certain patients may actually feel their depression worsen for the first week or so. Antidepressant medications are *not* addictive and do not generally give instantaneous relief. It usually takes about two weeks for an antidepressant medication to reach its full effect.

There are different classes of antidepressant medications, each with its own benefit and each with different side effects. One person may do better or tolerate the side effects better on a drug from one class over another.

Antidepressants have not yet been found to cause problems in infants of nursing mothers and are generally considered safe, but the nursing mother should be aware that the antidepressants do come through the milk, and studies have not been done on the long-term effect on infants.

There must also be an awareness that the FDA has approved these drugs only for short-term use. However, they tend to be prescribed for months and even years at a time. As yet, we do not know the long-term effects of these medications, and what the patient's cellular and neurotransmitter response is after long-term use.

Someone who is deeply depressed may need the assistance of medication to reach the point where she can become active in finding the cause of the depression.

My caution to those who choose to use and benefit from an antidepressant medication is to continue to look for the cause. Marie had multiple causes for her postpartum depression: hormonal imbalances, low thyroid, acid-base imbalance, excessive stress, sleep deprivation, and marital difficulties. Her depression did not completely lift until she was able to resolve the physical causes and work through many of the emotional causes. Remember that pain, both physical and emotional, is a message from the body trying to get our attention. If we suppress the pain, we may not hear the message and will lose an opportunity for growth. If you choose to take medication, continue to listen for the message that your body is sending you.

Nutrients, Herbs, and Homeopathic Remedies for Postpartum Depression

CAUTION: If you have been taking prescription drugs for depression or anxiety (antidepressants or tranquilizers) and want to stop them and change to natural remedies, you must not stop them suddenly. Sudden withdrawal from these drugs may cause physical problems, or may cause a psychological crisis, wherein the symptoms for which the medications were prescribed return in greater severity than originally. Consult your doctor and slowly reduce the dosage over a period of several weeks as you begin to take the natural remedies.

Vitamins and Minerals

I used to believe what I was taught in medical school, that we could get all the nutrition we needed from a good diet. I have since found, however, that it is very difficult for any of our diets to provide 100 percent of the essential nutrients at even the minimal

Recommended Daily Allowance (RDA) levels. Because of our poor eating habits and our overcooking of foods; because of poor soil nutrition, and the processing, radiating, and aging of foods, many of the nutrients in our foods are lost. Moreover, vitamin and mineral supplementation may become especially needed when the body and the brain are not functioning correctly, as can happen during the stresses of a woman's postpartum experience.

Multivitamin/mineral—I recommend to most of my patients to take a good multivitamin/mineral supplement, or an herbal supplement with high nutritional value.

Calcium—We all know that adequate calcium is needed for healthy bones, but calcium also aids in proper muscle and nerve function, sleeping, healthy blood vessel walls, muscle cramp prevention, and cancer protection. Calcium is calming to the system. The best calcium-containing foods are dark green vegetables, such as broccoli and spinach. If you are taking the mineral calcium, I would recommend about 800 mg a day of the chelated form, preferably in divided doses, along with trace minerals and vitamin D, which allow the body to utilize the calcium. Do not take calcium carbonate, which is what Tums are made of. Calcium carbonate is an antacid, reducing the amount of acid in your stomach. Your body needs adequate stomach acid to digest, absorb, and use the calcium (as well as many other nutrients and amino acids). The higher doses of calcium carbonate you take, the less acid you will have in your stomach, and your digestion and absorption of your food will be that much poorer. You would therefore need much higher doses of calcium to have any be absorbed.

Magnesium, potassium, and sodium—We have discussed magnesium in detail on page 264. Among its many benefits are its ability to protect us from muscle cramps, hormonal imbalances including PMS, menstrual cramps, heart attacks, preeclampsia of pregnancy, Alzheimer's, constipation, low blood sugar, diabetes, and osteoporosis. Again, a chelated source is best, because if magnesium is not absorbed well it will cause diarrhea. I recommend from 250 mg to 800 mg a day depending on the severity of your symptoms. Adequate potassium and sodium are also needed along with calcium and magnesium to maintain electrolyte and acid-base balance. Foods high in these minerals include oranges, beets, carrots, celery, cucumbers, okra, radishes, apples, cherries, strawberries, coconuts, figs, prunes, string beans, and spinach.

Vitamin B complex—Proper neurotransmitter function requires B vitamins for repair and maintenance. B-complex 50 will usually be adequate, although sometimes I will recommend higher doses of vitamin B$_6$ and folic acid. Consult your doctor or nutritionist for your specific needs. Whole grains, nutritional yeast, and meat are good sources of B vitamins.

Omega-3 and omega-6 fatty acids—Omega-3 fatty acids (fish and flaxseed oil) and omega-6 fatty acids (evening primrose and borage oil) are necessary for proper brain and nerve function, and have anti-inflammatory properties. They allow the body to make cholesterol, the building block of the sex and stress hormones. If you do not get enough fish in your diet, or do not eat enough natural vegetable fats, you may want to supplement with omega-3 and omega-6 fatty acids. Consider cooking with olive oil, sunflower seed oil, safflower oil, or grape-seed oil. Nuts and seeds are also a good source of healthy oils.

Trace minerals—Chromium assists in stabilizing blood sugar. Selenium is a potent antioxidant. Zinc, among other things, helps normalize appetite, especially in those with bulimia and anorexia nervosa. Multiple other trace minerals each have their function in the body and are necessary for proper acid-base balance.

Herbs to Use for Postpartum Depression

As with any supplements that you take while nursing or immediately after childbirth, please check with your doctor before using any of the following herbs. Review the possible use and dosages with your holistic physician.

Saint-John's-wort—Saint-John's-wort is the herb that has been subjected to the most studies of all herbs for depression. Studies from both the U.S. and Europe show that it can be as effective as Prozac, without as many of the side effects.

Valerian root—Valerian is a strong "nervine," or herb for the nerves, used for centuries to feed the nerves and calm the system from stress and nervous tension. It aids in relaxing the body for sleep.

Skullcap—Skullcap is another nervine, feeding the nerves and calming where nervousness results from worry and conflict. It also calms the nerves going to the muscles.

Hops—Hops are both a stimulating and relaxing nervine. They increase heart action and circulation, yet calm and help induce sleep when one is experiencing nervous and excited mental conditions.

Herbal combinations—My favorite combinations are Dr. Christopher's MindTrac for depression, and Relax-Eze for anxiety.

Herbs for hormonal imbalance—These herbs are discussed on page 255.

Homeopathic Remedies for Postpartum Depression

Homeopathic remedies are micro-doses of natural substances. A simplified explanation of the theory of homeopathy is that if a substance causes a symptom in a high dose, it will resolve that symptom in a micro-dose. The best way to use homeopathy in the case of postpartum depression is to visit a good classical homeopathic physician and receive a constitutional treatment (treating the whole person, not just the depression). These are some of the remedies that a homeopathic physician might consider. The names of the remedies are in Latin. The words written in bold are called "keynotes," and are generally integral to the symptoms, being indicators of the appropriate remedy.

Sepia—Consider sepia when the mother **does not bond with the baby**. She does not want to nurse or care for the baby, though unless the depression is very severe she will continue to do so anyway. She appears **indifferent** to the infant. She is easily angered and very irritable. She is usually **exhausted** by the end of the day, though exercise may make her feel better. She is also indifferent to her husband. She has a loss of energy and motivation, and a loss of sexual interest. She may gain weight rapidly following childbirth. The mother who could use sepia may feel unappreciated and used. She may have other children or a career and she doesn't want the responsibility of a new baby. She may blame and resent her husband for the pregnancy. She is frequently constipated and may have back pain.

Ignatia—Consider using ignatia if the mother's depression is due to **acute grief or a great disappointment** over some aspect of the labor or delivery, including premature birth, birth defects, cesarean section, difficulty nursing, or even the death of the infant. Whatever the cause, the mother had unfulfilled expectations and is deeply disappointed and many times feels guilty over the results. She may have wide mood swings, laughing at one moment and **weeping bitterly** the next. She generally has difficulty sleeping because of her grief or disappointment. She may sigh all the time.

Kali carbonicum—The woman who would benefit from kali carbonicum is **very irritable** and does not want to be touched. She is also hypersensitive to pain and noise. She is very **confused,** not knowing what is wrong, what she wants, or what to do with herself, and gives up trying. She becomes very depressed with much crying.

China officinalis—This remedy should be considered if the mother has lost a lot of blood during or after delivery. The depression may first be due to anemia from **loss of blood,** and then continue with nervous irritability, anxiety, or even hallucinations. She may be suicidal. There may be periodic fevers. She may be indifferent to others around her, with symptoms similar to those calling for sepia.

Natrum muriaticum—The mother who may benefit from this remedy has a sad, **brooding** depression in which she withdraws and

becomes worse when she is comforted or consoled. Life seems futile, and she is resigned to her condition, especially if there are marital problems and divorce does not seem to be an option, or any other situation in which she feels trapped. She may have undergone something that should have caused extreme grief, but she shut down emotionally and never worked through the grief. She may not be able to cry.

Arsenicum album—Consider this remedy if the mother becomes extremely insecure during her depression and does not want to be alone. She feels she cannot handle the baby, or even life, on her own. She is **full of fears and worries,** especially at night. She fears death but may be suicidal, which increases her fear. She is very **restless,** and may be frequently thirsty.

Aurum metallicum—This remedy benefits mothers who are deeply depressed and are strongly considering **suicide.** This woman is more likely to commit suicide than other women who may consider it but would never carry it through. *(Remember, anyone considering suicide should immediately seek help from a doctor, or call the suicide hotline at 1-800-SUICIDE.)* The mother feels totally worthless and unfit to live, knowing that all would be better without her. She may be oversensitive to noise, confusion, and excitement, which may send her into deeper depression. This mother may have experienced depression in the past, especially in the winter. She may tend to be a perfectionist and put high value on what she accomplishes. She may be very religious, praying continually.

Calcarea carbonica—This remedy is for postpartum depression in the **overworked, overwhelmed** woman who takes on too many responsibilities and has trouble saying no to people. She finds it hard to delegate responsibilities to others and never asks for help. She may fear that she is going crazy. She eventually loses interest in anything, including herself, and may become unkempt. She may have insomnia and constipation.

Veratrum album—Consider this remedy for the mother who suffered a complete mental and physical **collapse** following childbirth, usually brought on by some shock during childbirth. She may refuse to see a doctor for fear he or she will harm her. She can become manic-depressive, violent, and abusive. She may have periods where she refuses to speak. She is cold both emotionally and physically.

Pulsatilla—This mother will have wide **mood swings.** Her feelings are hurt at the slightest provocation, and she will **cry easily.** She becomes **needy and clingy,** demanding frequent attention, and others feel obligated to come to her rescue.

Ways to Increase Endorphin Levels

Each of the following activities has been shown to increase a person's endorphin levels and improve mood.

Laugh—Marie said that even though work was stressful for her, it also saved her, because she could laugh there. She felt that this laughing was what kept her from getting worse than she was. After laughing, she felt she could carry on for one more day. That was one of the reasons she wanted this book to be funny. If she could make you laugh, you would begin to feel better already. Laughing increases endorphin levels and improves the immune system.

Listen to music—Music can soothe and lift the soul like nothing else. The right music can clear the mind and heal the heart. Music has been found to be therapeutic in both physical and mental illnesses. It has been shown to improve brain function in children with learning disabilities. I consider music to be a form of vibrational medicine, if we find the music that is the right vibration for us.

Exercise—Exercise has been shown to increase serotonin and endorphin levels. Any kind of body motion will do. Walk, run, do aerobics, lift weights, play sports, run up and down stairs, or just turn on the radio and dance. Find something you enjoy doing, because you won't do it if you don't enjoy it. If you don't have an hour, do something for a half hour. If you don't have a half hour, do something for ten minutes. Any amount of good body motion will make a difference. Our bodies were made to move. If we stop moving, they become rusty, like the Tin Man, and don't want to move anymore. So take time to oil your joints and start moving again.

Do something you love to do—Often, as new mothers, we put everyone else before ourselves. It is hard to ignore a crying baby, and our partner's and other children's needs and wants fill our lives. But depression is a sign that something in our lives is out of order, and we need to occasionally have some time for ourselves. I consider myself like a car battery. I can give and give as long as I have something to build my own energy, but if I receive no energy for myself, my energy is soon gone, and I have nothing left to give. I have found that I have much more to give to my family if I am able to build myself up by doing something that I love to do. I don't consider this to be selfish but to be self-loving, and it allows me to give more love to others.

Dealing with Emotional Problems

How do we deal with emotional problems that are adding to our depression? There is no one way that works for all of us. The following are some possibilities that you may consider.

Counseling—Counseling has been shown to be as effective as antidepressant medication in resolving postpartum depression. However, there are many different types of counselors and many different methods of counseling. How do you choose the best counselor for you? You can start by asking friends and acquaintances for recommendations. You may wish to utilize referral services sponsored by cities, churches, or other organizations. Once you go to a counselor, personalities and/or beliefs may clash, so if you do not feel comfortable with him or her, leave and go to a different one. Most ethical counselors would not want to work with someone who feels uncomfortable with them. Do what Marie says and follow your intuition.

Self-help books—There are many books on the market that can assist women in dealing with the issues that face them. Look at the list of recommended reading at the back of this book.

Emotional work—There are many practitioners who use techniques that they may term "emotional work." Among them are osteopathic physicians and other body-work practitioners who find that emotions are stored in the body's muscles and tissues, and that when these are worked on, emotional release can occur. These techniques worked well for Marie.

Prayer—Studies have shown that religious practices and prayer have a very positive effect on healing.

Postpartum depression is a treatable condition. Help is available. No longer do women need to remain silent or feel embarrassed about their dark feelings during this time with their new infant. Speak up about your feelings and seek help. As you gain the courage to seek assistance for your condition, you will be increasing the awareness of the problem of postpartum depression in your community. You are not alone. Thousands of women are experiencing the same feelings you are. By finding and treating the physical and emotional causes of PPD, each mother can learn to find again the joy that life has to offer.

Appendix

SUICIDE HOTLINE

Suicide Crisis Center
1-800-SUICIDE
1-800-784-2433
http://suicidehotlines.com

POSTPARTUM DEPRESSION RESOURCES

Depression After Delivery
P.O. Box 278
Belle Mead, NJ 08502
(800) 944-4PPD (908) 575-9121
www.behavenet.com/dadinc

"MotherShare" chat room
www.members.nbci.com/Postpartum/chat.html

Postpartum Depression Bulletin Board
http://boards. parentsplace.com/messages/get/pppostdepression
71.html

Postpartum Education for Parents
(Provides publications and educational support)
P.O. Box 6154
Santa Barbara, CA 93160
www.sbpep.org

Postpartum Support International
(Directory of support groups, information, research,
publications, and web links)
www.chss.iup.edu/postpartum

Support for Fathers
(Information for men whose partners suffer with PPD)
www.pndinfo.co.uk

Washington's Family First (breast-feeding support)
5530 Wisconsin Ave., Suite 1136
Chevy Chase, MD 20815
www.levon-line.com/breastfeeding.html

NATURAL HORMONE RESOURCES

Compounding Pharmacies

ApotheCure
13720 Midway Road, Suite 109
Dallas, TX 75244
(800) 969-6610 Fax (800) 687-5252
www.apothecure.com

International Academy of Compounding Pharmacists
(Referrals for your area)
P.O. Box 1365
Sugarland, TX 77487
(800) 972-4227 Fax (281) 495-0602
www.compassnet.com/iacp

Jolley's Corner Pharmacy
1676 East 1300 South
Salt Lake City, UT 84105
(801) 582-1999

Professional Compounding Centers of America, Inc.
(800) 331-2498 Fax (800) 874-5760
www.thecompounders.com

Stewarts Plaza Pharmacy
3153 North Canyon Road
Provo, UT 84604
(801) 377-2002

Women's International Pharmacy
5708 Monona Drive
Madison, WI 53716
(800) 279-5708

Sources for Doctors Who Prescribe Natural Hormones

American College for Advancement in Medicine
23121 Verdugo Drive, Suite 204
P.O. Box 3427
Laguna Hills, CA 92654
(800) 532-3688 Fax (949) 455-9679
www.acam.org for physician referrals

Freedom Center for Advanced Medicine
Dennis W. Remington, M.D.
Judith S. Moore, D.O.
1675 N. Freedom Blvd., #11-E
Provo, UT 84604
(800) 373-8500
www.freedommedcenter.com

Sources for Natural Progesterone

There are many progesterone creams available, but many do not contain significant enough amounts of progesterone to create a change in your hormone levels. Make sure the product you use contains at least 400 mg of progesterone per ounce of cream. The following products have adequate amounts of progesterone, though there are many others.

Karuna Corp. (PhytoGest cream and PureGest gel)
42 Digital Dr., Suite 7
Novato, CA 94949
(888) 749-8643
www.kevalahealth.com

Transitions for Health, Inc. (Pro-Gest)
621 SW Alder, Suite 900
Portland, OR 97205
(800) 888-6814
www.transitionsforhealth.com

The above compounding pharmacies also can supply natural progesterone.

LABORATORY TESTING FOR SPECIALIZED FUNCTIONAL TESTING: SEX HORMONES, STRESS HORMONES, ALLERGIES, THYROID, AND YEAST

Aeron Life Cycles Laboratories
1933 Davis Street, Suite 310
San Leandro, CA 94577
(800) 631-7900 Fax (510) 729-0383
www.aeron.com

Antibody Assay Laboratories
1715 E. Wilshire, #715
Santa Ana, CA 92705
(800) 522-2611 Fax (714) 543-2034
www.antibodyassay.com

Diagnos-Techs, Inc., Clinical and Research Laboratory
6620 S. 192nd Place, Bldg. J
Kent, WA 98032
(800) 878-3787 Fax (425) 251-9520
www.diagnostechs.com

Great Smokies Diagnostic Laboratory
63 Zillicoa St.
Asheville, NC 28801
(800) 522-4762 Fax (828) 252-9303
www.gsdl.com

Meridian Valley Clinical Laboratories
515 West Harrison St., Suite 9
Kent, WA 98032
(800) 234-6825 Fax (253) 859-1135
www.meridianvalleylab.com

MetaMetrix Clinical Laboratory
5000 Peachtree Industrial Blvd.
Norcross, Georgia 30071
(800) 221-4640 Fax (770) 441-2237
www.metametrix.com

SpectraCell Laboratories, Inc.
(Tests for nutrient deficiencies)
515 Post Oak Blvd., Suite 830
Houston, TX 77027
(800) 227-5227 Fax (713) 621-3234
www.spectracell.com

HOMEOPATHIC RESOURCES

Referrals for Homeopathic Physicians

International Foundation for Homeopathy
2366 Eastlake Ave East, Suite 325
Seattle, WA 98102
(206) 324-8230

National Center for Homeopathy
(Directory of homeopathic practitioners and study groups)
801 North Fairfax Street, Suite 306
Alexandria, VA 22314
(703) 548-7790 Fax (703) 548-7792
www.homeopathic.org

The Homeopathic Academy of Naturopathic Physicians
P.O. Box 69565
Portland, OR 97201
(503) 795-0579 Fax (503) 829-8541

Homeopathic Pharmacies

Boericke & Tafel, Inc.
1011 Arch St.
Philadelphia, PA 19107
(800) 276-2870 (East Coast)
(800) 876-9505 (West Coast)

Boiron-Bornemann, Inc.
98C Cochran St.
Simi Valley, CA 93065
(800) 258-8823 Fax (800) 999-4373

Dolisos, Inc.
3014 Rigel Avenue
Las Vegas, NV 89102
(800) 365-4767
www.dolisos.com

Hahnemann Medical Pharmacy
1940 4th Street
San Rafael, CA 94901
(888) 472-6422
www.hahnemannpharmacy.com

Standard Homeopathic Company
210 West 131st Street, Box 61067
Los Angeles, CA 90061
(800) 624-9659 (800) 992-9659 (California)
Fax (310) 516-8579
www.hylands.com

Homeopathic Literature

Homeopathic Educational Services
2124 Kittredge St., #71Q
Berkeley, CA 94704
(510) 649-0294 (800) 359-9051
www.homeopathic.com

HERBAL RESOURCES

American Association of Naturopathic Physicians
8201 Greensboro Dr., Suite 300
McLean, VA 22102
(703) 610-9000
www.naturopathic.org

Dr. Christopher's Original Herbal Formulas
Herbs First (Herbs, books, tapes, videos, and education)
501 West 965 North, Suite 3
Orem, UT 84057
Fax (801) 818-4155
www.herbsfirst.com

Murdock Pharmaceuticals, Inc./Nature's Way
(Herbs and nutrients)
10 Mountain Springs Parkway
Springville, UT 84663
(800) 962-8873 Fax (801) 489-1700
www.naturesway.com

NuLegacy International, Inc.
(Herbs, nutrients, and glandulars)
1815 North 1120 West
Provo, UT 84604-1180
(888) 205-3422 Fax (801) 356-0737
www.nulegacy.com
www.legacyofhealth.com
   (Note: This company is a network marketing company. You
may order retail or choose to join and order wholesale. Either
way, the company has agreed that a portion of all orders originating from this book will go to the Foundation for the
Advancement of Integrated Medicine.)

Pain & Stress Center
(Anxiety Control, with GABA, nutrients, and herbs)
5282 Medical Drive, #160
San Antonio, TX 78229
(800) 669-2256
www.painstresscenter.com

Phyto Pharmica
(FemTone herbal phytohormonal product)
Green Bay, WI 54311
www.phytopharmica.com

Standard Process
(Herbs, nutrients, and glandulars)
1200 West Royal Lee Drive
P.O. Box 904
Palmyra, WI 53156-0904
(800) 848-5061
www.standardprocess.com

Young Living Essential Oils
(Pure herbal oils, aromatherapy)
250 South Main Street
Payson, UT 84651
(800) 350-5042 Fax (800) 883-9576
www.youngliving.com
   (Note: This company is a network marketing company. You may order retail or choose to join and order wholesale. Either way, the company has agreed that a portion of all orders originating from this book will go to the Foundation for the Advancement of Integrated Medicine.)

NUTRITIONAL RESOURCES

American Association of Nutritional Consultants
302 E. Wiona Avenue
Warsaw, IN 46580
(888) 828-2262 Fax (219) 267-2614
www.healthkeepers.net (for practitioner referrals)

American College for Advancement in Medicine
23121 Verdugo Drive, Suite 204
P.O. Box 3427
Laguna Hills, CA 92654
(800) 532-3688 Fax (949) 455-9679
www.acam.org (for physician referrals)

Price-Pottenger Nutrition Foundation
P.O. Box 2614
La Mesa, CA 91943
(619) 574-7763 Fax (619) 574-1314
www.price-pottenger.org (for Healthcare practitioner referrals)

MENTAL HEALTH AND EMOTIONAL
WORK INFORMATION

American Psychiatric Association/Division of Public Affairs,
Department HH
(Referrals to certified psychiatrists)
1400 K Street NW
Washington, DC 20005
(202) 682-6000 Fax (202) 682-6850
www.psych.org

Applied Psycho-Neurobiology
American Academy of Neural Therapy
(206) 749-9967 or e-mail at aant@neuraltherapy.com
www.neuraltherapy.com

Emotional Stress Integration
BioMeridian International, contact Dorothy Sudweeks
12411 S. 265 W., Suite F
Draper, UT 84020
(888) 224-2377 Fax (801) 501-7518
www.biomeridian.com

International Association of Counselors and Therapists
(Licensed or certified counselors or mental health therapists
with strong interest in complementary therapies and approaches)
10915 Bonita Beach Road SE, #1101
Bonita Springs, FL 34135
(941) 498-9710 Fax (941) 498-1215
www.iact.org

The National Association for Holistic Aromatherapy
2000 2nd Avenue, Suite 206
Seattle, WA 98121
(888) ASK-NAHA Fax (206) 770-5915
www.naha.org

NAET Research Foundation
(Emotional work in association with allergy treatment)
6714 Beach Blvd.
Buena Park, CA 90621
(714) 523-8900 Fax (714) 523-3068
www.naet.com

Neuro-Emotional Technique (NET)
The ONE Foundation
1991 Village Park Way, Suite 201A
Encinitas, CA 92024
www.onefoundation.org

OSTEOPATHIC MANIPULATION, CRANIAL OSTEOPATHY

American Academy of Osteopathy
(Osteopathic physicians who specialize in osteopathic
manipulative treatment)
3500 DePauw Blvd., Suite 1080
Indianapolis, IN 46268-1136
(317) 879-1881 Fax (317) 879-0563
www.academyofosteopathy.org

American Osteopathic Association
142 East Ontario St.
Chicago, IL 60611
(800) 621-1773 Fax (312) 202-8200
www.am-osteo-assn.org

Cranial Academy
(Osteopathic physicians who have specialized training in
cranial osteopathy)
8202 Clearvista Parkway, #9D
Indianapolis, IN 46256
(317) 594-0411 Fax (317) 594-9299
E-mail: CranAcad@aol.com
(Send 55 cents and a self-addressed stamped envelope
 for a list of physicians in your state.)

Osteopathic Center for Children
4135 54th Place
San Diego, CA 92105
(619) 583-7611 Fax (619) 583-0296
www.osteopathic-ctr-4child.org/contacts

MASSAGE THERAPISTS AND OTHER BODY WORKERS

International Association of Healthcare Practitioners
(Massage and other therapists trained in craniosacral therapy, vis-
ceral manipulation, lymph drainage, neuromuscular therapy, etc.)
11211 Prosperity Farms Rd., Suite D325
Palm Beach Gardens, FL 33410
(800) 311-9204 Fax (561) 622-4771

The Trager Institute
21 Locust Avenue
Mill Valley, CA 94941
(415) 388-2688 Fax (415) 388-2710
www.trager.com

HIGH RESOLUTION MICROSCOPY

The Bradford Research Institute/American Biologics
1180 Walnut Ave.
Chula Vista, CA 91911
(800) 227-4473
www.americanbiologics.com

Enderlein Enterprises
P.O. Box 11510
Prescott, AZ 86304
(602) 439-7977 Fax (888) 439-7980
www.pleomorphic.com

NuLife Sciences
1321D Commerce St.
Petaluma, CA 94954
(707)781-9557 Fax (707) 781-9559
www.crl.com/-nulife

Recommended Reading

1. Bass, Ellen and Laura Davis. *Beginning to Heal: A First Book for Survivors of Child Sexual Abuse*. New York: Harperperennial Library, 1993.

2. Benson, Herbert. *The Relaxation Response*. New York: Avon, 1990.

3. Chopra, Deepak. *Quantum Healing: Exploring the Frontiers of Mind/Body Medicine*. New York: Bantam, 1989.

4. Fulford, Robert C., D.O. *Dr. Fulford's Touch of Life: The Healing Power of the Natural Life Force*. New York: Pocket Books, 1996.

5. Gawain, Shakti. *Creative Visualization*. New York: Bantam, 1982.

6. Hauri, Peter and Shirley Linde. *No More Sleepless Nights: A Proven Program to Conquer Insomnia*. New York: Wiley, 1996.

7. Hay, Louise L. *You Can Heal Your Life*. Carlsbad, CA: Hay House, 1987.

8. Moore, Judith, D.O. *Healing from the Heart: The Inherent Power to Heal from Within*. Provo, UT: Vitality House, 2001.

9. Myss, Caroline. *Why People Don't Heal and How They Can*. Nevada City, CA: Harmony Books, 1997.

10. Northrup, Christiane. *Women's Bodies, Women's Wisdom*. New York: Bantam, 1994.

11. Remington, Dennis, M.D. and Barbara H. Swasey. *Back to Health: A Comprehensive Medical and Nutritional Yeast Control Program*. Provo, UT: Vitality House, 1989.
12. Woodman, Marion. *Pregnant Virgin: A Process of Psychological Transformation*. Toronto, CAN: Inner City Books, 1988.